Rethink
Chronic
Pain

〰

DR. GAÉTAN BROUILLARD

TRANSLATED BY DAVID WARRINER

〰〰

Relieve Suffering, Heal Your Body, Own Your Health

Rethink Chronic Pain

〰〰

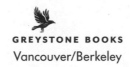

GREYSTONE BOOKS

Vancouver/Berkeley

20 21 22 23 24   5 4 3 2 1

Greystone Books Ltd.
greystonebooks.com

Cataloguing data available from Library and Archives Canada
ISBN 978-1-77164-463-1 (pbk.)
ISBN 978-1-77164-464-8 (epub)

Copy editing by Paula Ayer
Proofreading by Alison Strobel
Cover design by Belle Wuthrich and Fiona Siu
Text design by Nayeli Jimenez
Illustrations by Jean-François Vachon
Medical review by Dr. Tanya Cabrita

Printed and bound in Canada on ancient-forest-friendly paper by Friesens

This work reflects the ideas and opinions of the author. It aims to provide useful information on the topics covered in these pages. Neither the author nor the publisher is offering medical, health, or other professional services in this book. Before putting the suggestions in this book into practice or drawing conclusions from them, readers should consult their general practitioner or another competent health professional. The author and the publisher are not responsible for any liability, damage, loss, or risk, whether personal or otherwise, suffered as a result of the direct or indirect use or application of any element of the contents of this work. Patient names have been changed to protect privacy.

Greystone Books gratefully acknowledges the Musqueam, Squamish, and Tsleil-Waututh peoples on whose land our office is located.

Greystone Books thanks the Canada Council for the Arts, the British Columbia Arts Council, the Province of British Columbia through the Book Publishing Tax Credit, and the Government of Canada for supporting our publishing activities.

Canad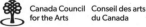

Contents

IIIIIIIIIIIIIIIIIIIIIIIIIIIIIIIIIIIIIIIIIIIIIIIII

Introduction

||||||||||||||||||||||||||||||||||||||||||||||||||||||||||

Pain is universal, and to some degree, it's a part of our daily lives. Whether it's the dull ache of a small dental cavity or the intense shooting pain of a broken bone, pain is a fact of life, and it always has been. Most pain comes and goes, but when it persists—for longer than three to six months, by definition—it becomes chronic. Chronic pain affects more than 20 percent of us at some point in our lives, and sometimes it lasts for the rest of our lives. Pain is the number one reason people visit the doctor's office, and it's also the main motivation for seeking medical help for chronic conditions. It's a bigger problem in today's society than we might think. I have encountered people whose pain was so unbearable they were near the brink of suicide.

After more than forty years of medical practice focused on relieving human suffering, I felt a duty to help people in pain understand what they're going through. *Why me?* they ask. *Why am I trapped in this vicious cycle of pain? It seems so unfair.*

I also felt that I should share my knowledge by offering people simple tools to help relieve the various ailments that are so frequent on this great planet of ours, where modern medicine is still very much experimenting when it comes to explaining and treating the pervasive presence of pain.

I'll be the first to admit that pain is not something that's easy to wrap our heads around, and it's even harder to live with. Pain may be inevitable at some point or another, so it's important for us to learn how to break free from its grip insofar as possible, using techniques that are often simple and without undesirable side effects. Ideally, we should also become more aware and mindful of the distressing reality of chronic pain, because if we don't, it can easily ruin our lives.

We might not realize it, but we often play a significant part in the genesis of our pain. The good news is that we can also play an active part in overcoming our pain, or at least relieving it. Let's not forget that we are always the co-creators of our own lives. As the American author James Baldwin said, "Not everything that is faced can be changed, but nothing can be changed until it is faced."

QUALITY MEDICINE THAT PUTS PEOPLE FIRST

This book offers a general overview and a fresh outlook for anyone suffering from pain. We'll explore some of the latest treatments that are recognized in North America and around the world, and we'll offer ways to understand the pain that can sometimes be hard to separate ourselves from.

Science has now proven just how important a role our lifestyle can play in the quality of our health,[1] and also, unfortunately, what a critical factor it can be in the emergence of many of the chronic illnesses and types of pain afflicting us today.[2] It's time to embrace an approach to medicine that doesn't just prescribe treatment for pain and illness, but that also probes the cause of the conditions that ail us.

My preferred approach is **functional medicine**, which aims to treat the whole person by tracing imbalances in the body back to their source. Functional medicine works at every level of our being.[3] It is intuitive and based on knowledge of all biochemical interconnections. Functional medicine treats the person, not the illness. It is both inclusive and integrative, because it embraces treatments using supplements, plants, and pharmaceuticals as needed. It also advocates for a true model of preventive health. We're not talking about the kind of prevention that consists of having X-rays and blood tests done at your annual checkup, but the kind that involves leading a healthy lifestyle and taking other prophylactic measures to steer clear of illness. With functional medicine, the focus is on health, not on illness. This approach touches on every aspect of prevention and promotes the use of recognized treatments. It embraces the synthesis of complementary and integrative medicine for the well-being of patients and society itself. Here's what the World Health Organization has to say about it: "Patients whose GP has additional [complementary and alternative medicine training have] lower healthcare costs and mortality rates [...]. The lower costs result from fewer hospital stays and fewer prescription drugs."[4]

We must stop being so resistant to complementary health approaches. After all, these treatments are widely recognized and deliver great benefits to the significant numbers of patients who try them. Now is the time for us to stand up and take our health in hand. This is a message that speaks for itself, and it's what I've been striving to convey to my patients for more than forty years.

HOW I CAME TO SPECIALIZE IN TREATING PAIN

I started my career as a doctor at Montreal's Maisonneuve-Rosemont Hospital, in one of the busiest emergency rooms in Canada that deals with some of the most serious cases there are. Pain is everywhere you look in the ER, and emergency doctors have no choice but to treat it. That duty extends to every physician, even outside the ER, because nearly 75 percent of a family doctor's work consists of treating pain. Pain is therefore a normal part of medical practice.

Back pain was one of the most common complaints my colleagues and I encountered in the emergency room. Whether they were the victims of a workplace accident, an unfortunate fall, a failed attempt to lift something heavy, or simply the slightest false move at home, patients would often arrive by ambulance, their pain so intense they couldn't move.

At some point I realized how limited the approach of traditional Western medicine was when it came to relieving and treating this kind of pain. Of course, we had access to painkillers and muscle relaxants, but these drugs took time to kick in, not to mention that they couldn't completely control the pain. And any spasmodic pain (which causes cramps) or neurological pain (connected to nerve damage) that ensued would often take a long time to fade away. What's more, we often saw patients returning several weeks or months later, complaining of a problem we thought we had solved. Why were these recurrences so frequent? Because we hadn't identified what was at the root of the complaint. We had only treated the symptoms, and not the source of the problem.

Once I started seeing patients in private practice, I came up against many more of these complex cases that conventional medicine struggled so hard to treat. Many of my colleagues in the same practice would grow frustrated after a few months at the complexity of the cases we found ourselves treating. But I refused to give up and accept that there was nothing we could do to help these suffering patients. And so I started looking to alternative approaches in the United States and Europe for insight, and for complementary knowledge and tools that would enable me to suggest different solutions—ones that were focused on the patient and the underlying causes of their illness, that had proven themselves to work elsewhere, but that patients here had never tried.

The more of these new techniques and treatments I learned about, the more challenging and complex a clientele I started to see in my practice. In fact, the stories I heard from new patients would often go something along the lines of: "Doctor, I've tried everything to get to the bottom of this. I've seen lots of different specialists, tried so many different approaches, and ten years later, here I am, still with the same problem."

WHAT I LEARNED FROM MY WIFE'S BACK PAIN

My wife, Carole, was one of those people for whom I found myself looking for solutions. When I first met her, she had been suffering from back pain for several years, since a water-skiing accident she had when she was fifteen years old. At the time, she had been prescribed several weeks of rest, as well as painkillers, muscle relaxants, and intensive physiotherapy treatments. Over time, the pain gradually faded, but it would return intermittently. When the pain came back, it was uncomfortable, but bearable.

The pain worsened when Carole was twenty-three years old. We had been married for a year at that point. The pain grew even more stubborn and intense after our first child came along, and picking up and carrying the baby only aggravated the situation. Carole's pain in the back was also accompanied by what we commonly refer to as sciatic pain, which started in the right lumbar region, radiated into her buttock and the back of her thigh, and continued all the way down to her calf and foot.

A medical examination had shown that a nerve root was being compressed by a disc in her lumbar spine. First, we turned to medication, physiotherapy, and various forms of spinal traction, as these were the usual medical treatments at the time.

At one point, a neurosurgeon decided to operate and remove the damaged disc to free the sciatic nerve that was causing so much pain in the leg. In the weeks that followed, the pain went away—but only partially. Carole was still vulnerable and the slightest effort could cause her spasmodic pain, leaving her so incapacitated she could barely walk.

Determined to find a solution to my wife's pain, I started to turn to lesser-known forms of medicine, such as massage techniques, which led to some interesting gains in relieving the pain, restoring movement, and building muscle strength. One day, Carole asked me what I thought about acupuncture and whether it might help.

Thirty-five years ago, in our part of Canada, acupuncture was far from being as common and recognized as it is today. I told her I knew nothing about it, but when I looked into it, I figured a practice that was thousands of years old must be solidly grounded if it had stood the test of time, even surviving through periods of Chinese history when its use had been banned. At Carole's urging, I signed up to start studying at the Acupuncture Foundation of Canada, and my wife later became my first patient.

These various methods brought considerable relief to Carole, to the point where her pain had almost completely disappeared. However, she remained vulnerable to relapse. Her treatment was still lacking something that would give her more strength, given how weak the surgery had made her ligaments.

SOME PROMISING NEW TECHNIQUES

At that time—the early 1980s—a British orthopedist by the name of James Cyriax came to the United States to train doctors. The remarkable thing about this specialist was that he had moved away from his work as an orthopedic surgeon in favor of developing techniques to manipulate the spine and joints.[5] This struck me as highly unusual, since in our part of Canada there was no such thing as a physician who manipulated patients' spines and joints. This doctor clearly knew what he was doing, however, since he had been treating a number of celebrity patients, including members of the British royal family!

As a general practitioner who wanted to treat muscle and joint pain, I was immediately drawn to this form of orthopedic medicine, which promised to avoid, or at the very least defer, surgical intervention where possible. And so every year I would travel down to the United States four or five times to train with Dr. Cyriax's team and to study functional medicine, in addition to working my regular shifts in the ER and outpatient clinic and seeing patients in private practice.

Toward the end of his orthopedic practice, Dr. Cyriax also developed a range of targeted injection techniques on the strength of his clinical experience. Still wanting to help Carole as best I could, I signed up for the seminars Dr. Cyriax and his team were presenting.

In the end, it was precisely this type of injection that provided Carole with complete relief from her pain once and for all. I went on to make this injection technique my specialty. **Prolotherapy**, as it is known, consists of injecting reparative substances into the tissue. We'll explore this in detail in Chapter 6.

In the months that followed my encounter with Dr. Cyriax, I also spent time with another great physician, Dr. Robert Maigne, who was the head of the department of rheumatology and orthopedics at the Hôtel-Dieu de Paris. Dr. Maigne excelled in the "small world" of manual osteopathic medicine. Thanks to him, I was able to broaden my experience in the field of manual treatment and injection therapy.[6]

As I applied simple techniques to complex and chronic problems and saw how they could often be solved once and for all, my career path grew more and more interesting—so much so that my colleagues would refer patients to me who were not responding to the usual medications. Occasionally I was even able to put this new knowledge to use in the emergency room. As I had learned a number of spinal mobilization techniques, when I could see that the cause of the patient's pain was a spinal blockage, I was able to do manipulations, and as a result, often the patient could walk out of the hospital without any pain and without taking any medication at all. Through careful palpation, I was able to feel, for example, whether there was a blockage or restriction on one side, and restore movement through manipulations. The results were often astonishing, especially for neck and back problems, but also for ankle and knee injuries.

THE DANGERS OF SELF-DIAGNOSIS

Here's one of the lessons I learned from these great doctors that I have always found useful, in both the ER and in my own practice: don't judge a book by its cover, because the source of the pain isn't necessarily where the patient says it hurts. That's why, dear readers, I would like to say a word of caution about the dangers of self-diagnosis, especially in these times when the internet seems to have an answer—and another, contradictory answer—for everything!

To avoid waiting for hours in the emergency room, it can be tempting for many of us to surf the web quickly in search of an easy fix for an ailment, even if we're not exactly medical experts. However, self-diagnosing an ailment can do more harm than good. It's easy to be lured down a rabbit hole by many websites out there. The more worried we are—about a serious illness, for example—the more likely we are to throw caution to the wind and believe the first opinion that promises recovery. Dr. Yves Robert, chief executive officer and secretary of the Collège des médecins du Québec, offers some food for thought: "People are blind to the commercial interests of the sites they visit, many of which are run by some less than scrupulous companies selling products that seem too good to be true. For people whose health is seriously compromised, the internet is a land of miracle promises full of questionable sites that play on their hope for a cure and their dreams of security."[7]

Health is a major issue, and there will never be a shortage of websites popping up to reassure those who are suffering. Although some of these can be reliable sources of information, the effectiveness of self-diagnosis will always be debatable. There's still no substitute for a visit to your doctor or another health professional. It's the best way to avoid any unfortunate consequences. (To prove this point, something you might not be aware of is that a sudden and intense headache may be an early indicator of a brain aneurysm.) Obviously, it's in our nature to seek answers to our questions, and there's nothing wrong with that. By all means, do a little research, but then talk to a pain specialist about what you've found. It's only by working together and exchanging knowledge that we can tap into the true power of medicine.

Pain is a complex thing to treat, even for doctors who are trained to do so. Sometimes it takes a number of experts to find a solution to a patient's chronic pain. Don't let pain ruin your quality of life, however, and don't let it be incapacitating. Don't give up too soon on trying to get well again. Even if you have seen several doctors and therapists already, I encourage you to keep looking. I hope that this book can help you to break free of the grip of suffering and develop a better understanding of any pain that persists. You'll find lots of tips in here that might just change your life. Let me be your guide throughout this book and help you find a sense of well-being you probably haven't felt for a long time. It's time to make a change.

CHAPTER 1

Understanding Pain

||||||||||||||||||||||||||||||||||||||||||||||||||||||||||||||||||||

Man is a pupil, pain is his teacher.

ALFRED DE MUSSET

S INCE WE'RE GOING to be talking about pain throughout this book, let's start by defining what it is. Pain is a manifestation of an imbalance in your body that you feel as an unpleasant sensation. Think of it as an alarm going off to warn you of a danger or a threat to your physical or emotional body. (That's right: pain can be psychological, too.) It's irritating, it's unwanted, and it can affect your quality of life. Pain creates a sense of unease and discomfort. But worst of all, pain isn't something you can see. It doesn't show up in a blood test or on an X-ray. And you can't show it to anyone else. Pain is something you feel and experience alone. That's why it can be so challenging to try to explain it to someone.

The *Merriam-Webster Dictionary* defines pain as "the physical feeling caused by disease, injury, or something that hurts the body." The definition also extends to psychological pain, citing "acute mental or emotional distress or suffering."

According to the International Association for the Study of Pain, pain is "an unpleasant sensory and emotional experience associated with actual or potential tissue damage."[1] Going by this particular definition, pain is never solely physical; the emotional aspect is always there, too. Pain, therefore, is a subjective thing, and we all feel it at different intensities depending on how sensitive we are.

Pain is considered to be *acute* if it is short-lived (though it can be very intense), or *chronic* if it recurs or persists for longer than three to six months (depending on who you ask). In many ways, pain can be a useful thing, because it essentially sounds the alarm and helps you to avoid doing any further damage to your body.

Keep reading, and you'll find out how pain has a cause, a source, and even a meaning.

Pain is necessary

Pain stems from a change in tissue. Thanks to your nervous system, your brain registers any change your body undergoes, and pain is the mechanism your body uses to tell you that something is wrong or out of the ordinary. Without this mechanism to sound the alarm, you wouldn't know something was happening that might pose a threat to your body or to one of your organs. Think of a burn as a simple example of this. If you put your hand on a hot stove, the searing pain you experience is your brain's way of telling you about the risk of damage to your hand. Your hand doesn't feel the pain; rather, receptors in your hand send signals to your brain, which decodes the sensation as pain. Before you even realize the stove is red-hot, you instinctively pull your hand away, because your nervous system immediately tells your bicep to contract.

Pain plays an essential role in alerting you to danger. Because of damage to sensitive nerve fibers, some people with chronic diabetes experience a decreased sensitivity to pain in their feet. As such, they might easily walk on hot coals or step on a nail without realizing the damage they're causing to their foot. This means they must be very careful to avoid hurting themselves. Ultimately, pain is a protection mechanism and a survival-instinct tool for your body, and you have your nervous system to thank for it.

The pain circuit

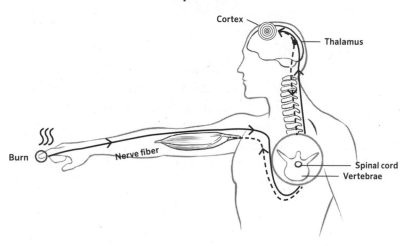

Cortex

Thalamus

Burn

Nerve fiber

Spinal cord

Vertebrae

Pain is personal

Most people's reaction to touching a hot stove would be to pull their hand away. However, in some situations, tolerance to pain can vary dramatically from one person to another. Think of a visit to the dentist's office, where it's easy to see the two extremes. Some people can have dental work done without any anesthetic at all, while others need to be heavily medicated to undergo the same procedure—and can find the pain so unbearable they might even pass out, especially once fear comes into play. Meanwhile, others may undergo a similar procedure that would usually require anesthetic with the help of hypnosis or acupuncture alone. Pain perception can vary tremendously depending on the person, their age, how accustomed they are to the feeling, how tired they are, and even their emotional state. Pain is therefore a very personal thing, and we can all experience different intensities of pain at different times.

Giving birth is another interesting example of how pain can vary radically from one person to another. While there are many factors involved in giving birth and some women no doubt have a more difficult experience than others, even given similar situations some women will find the pain unbearable, while others give birth seemingly easily and almost painlessly.

It seems there may also be a sociocultural dimension to the perception of pain. One thing that struck me when I went to work with the Innu in the northern Quebec town of Schefferville was the high pain resilience exhibited by some Indigenous people. I recall being able to perform some surgery—on adults and children alike—using only minimal local anesthetic, all very successfully. I found myself treating children who had ear infections with ruptured eardrums, but who complained of very little or no pain.

My few weeks as a locum in the far north soon came to an end, and before I left to catch my plane home to Montreal, I did the rounds one last time. All inpatients were receiving proper care and the emergency room was empty. All was calm as I prepared to thank the nurses and bid them farewell. Considering that, at that time, there was only one doctor for nearly four thousand people in the Schefferville area, the nurses there did a remarkable job and were highly talented. They would often diagnose patients and begin treatment in the middle of the night, saving the doctor precious hours of sleep. There are no roads to speak of into or out of this remote town, and back then it was only accessible by plane once a week, and sometimes only every two weeks.

Therefore I knew I had to leave in the next hour, on the same plane my replacement was flying in on. I was quite sad to be leaving, since I had enjoyed working there with the keen staff and friendly people in the town. It was at this point that Jade Shu Lee walked into the outpatient clinic at the Schefferville hospital. This young woman of Asian descent was expecting her first baby and presented with uterine contractions. She calmly told me her contractions were close together and that she was probably very close to giving birth. As I carried out a pelvic examination, I was astounded to see her cervix was already significantly dilated. I figured that she would be giving birth in a few hours and that the nurses, together with my replacement, would take care of her.

I performed another examination and realized that her cervix was fully dilated and that the uterine contractions were doing their job very well indeed. Yet my patient was remarkably cool, calm, and collected, displaying no signs of concern or suffering, even though this was her first child. She was alone, with no one to help her through the birth. I asked her how she was feeling and how severe the pain was. She told me she was fine and wasn't in any pain. It looked like she was carrying a big baby for such a petite frame. And so I administered an injection to anesthetize the perineum and performed an episiotomy—a small incision—to help ease the way for the baby and minimize tearing. Jade remained perfectly calm throughout all of this, never displaying any discomfort.

Everything progressed much quicker than I had expected. Jade's contractions were very efficient, and a little head soon appeared. We carried on a conversation the whole time and at no point did Jade show any sign of suffering. I was flabbergasted by such restraint in the face of pain, to the point where I wondered whether her neurons were wired differently from most people's! Before I knew it, Jade was holding her beautiful baby boy, full of life, in her arms.

I hadn't finished stitching up the episiotomy when a nurse ran over to tell me I had to leave right away, as the plane wouldn't wait. Obviously, I didn't want to leave my patient with a tear that I hadn't closed, but there was no arguing with the nurse, who was adamant that if I missed this plane, there wouldn't be another one for another week or two. I knew my colleague would be arriving at the hospital less than ten minutes later, since he was aboard the plane that had just landed.

Reluctantly, I explained to Jade that if it was all right with her, I would have to leave her to catch my plane, and that my colleague would be with her shortly to finish her stitches. She smiled and told me not to worry, joking that she was in good hands with the nurses anyway. As I left, to my great surprise there was no taxi waiting for me at the hospital entrance, but a police cruiser, which promptly raced off to the airport with lights blazing and sirens blaring. This was quite a surreal experience for me, since I was so used to seeing ambulances and police cars arriving at the emergency room, not leaving it. I boarded the plane just in time, my head spinning with thoughts of all the kind, generous people I had been able to help during my short time there.

Differences in individual pain tolerance are difficult to explain. Could it be that our perception of pain, which isn't purely physiological, also depends on our state of mind?

Do we learn to feel pain?

Many researchers have examined the question of pain perception. One notable example is Dr. Ronald Melzack,[2] whose work includes a study on dogs that were bred in an environment that had never exposed them to pain. Once they were fully grown, they reacted differently to injections than other animals, as if they didn't recognize the sensation of pain because they had never learned what it was. According to Dr. Melzack, pain depends as much on our experiences as on our instincts. This is interesting, because it suggests we also have the capacity to *unlearn* how to feel pain. Hypnosis has demonstrated how we can manipulate the sensation of pain by feeding our brain a different program than the one it knows. We'll look at the benefits of hypnosis in greater depth in Chapter 6, which is all about treating pain.

DO WE FEEL FEAR MORE THAN PAIN?

One important realization that research has brought to light is that the apprehension of pain can augment the sensation—it can even make it feel twice as intense. However, the opposite is also true. One of my patients used to faint whenever I injected his medication, so I started administering a drug that would prevent his blood pressure from dropping so that he could confront the pain. After two more of his shots, he was no longer afraid of fainting and realized the needles didn't actually hurt as much as he had remembered. In fact, his "needle pain" completely disappeared from then on.

I often have to be careful when someone accompanies a patient into my office for an injection. They sometimes have to leave because they feel faint at the sight of their friend getting an injection, even when the patient experiences no pain from the shot and keeps smiling the whole time!

The level of pain we feel—or the apprehension of that pain—bears no relation to the size of the person.

A patient of mine, a police officer who's six foot four and weighs nearly two hundred pounds, asked me to slot him in one day between two appointments because he was on duty and was in a hurry to get a shot to relieve himself from severe shoulder pain. I took my time administering the injection, only to see this giant of a man turn as white as a sheet and promptly pass out. He was in such a hurry when he walked into my office, but it took him nearly forty minutes to come to his senses and walk out again.

SOMETIMES WE FORGET IT HURTS

After a traffic accident, it's not uncommon for parents who have withstood fractures to keep moving long enough to help their children get out of the car—they're so focused on helping their injured children that they barely sense their own pain. The same phenomenon has been observed in terrorist attacks, when people injured in a bomb blast help others to safety. Once the danger has passed, they're amazed that they didn't feel the pain of a broken limb or a deep laceration. It's surprising to realize just how much our psyche can play tricks on us when it comes to pain. As much as we can suffer in anticipation of pain, we can seemingly just as well tame the sensation when something else monopolizes our attention.

THE PAIN—AND EUPHORIA—OF AN ATHLETE

Athletes competing in an event tend not to react much to pain. They'll keep on running even if their foot is hurting, or if they're out of breath and the intense effort is causing them chest pains. If they hurt their ankle on the final sprint while they're in the lead, they'll finish the race that will make them a champion, only collapsing in pain once they've crossed the finish line. Even then, they manage to get right back up again, because they won the race! As the medical team zeroes in to help, they'll say, "I really don't feel the pain that much, because I won." But if they had lost, they would likely have crumpled to the ground before the finish line, crippled by the pain.

Context, favorable or not, can influence our perception of the intensity of pain tremendously. Under the effect of a heavy dose of adrenaline, we simply don't feel it as much, especially as nature has given us endorphins—a morphine-like substance produced by the body—to neutralize the painful effects of an injury.[3] These endorphins, a type of neurotransmitter (page 37), are proteins secreted by our pituitary gland and hypothalamus during intense physical activity (such as a long run), pain, excitement, and even orgasm. In addition to their pain-relieving effects, endorphins can give athletes a feeling of joy and well-being during an intense and prolonged period of effort.

Be careful not to push yourself too hard with exhilarating extreme sports, however, in case you end up having to forgo exercise completely due to repeated injury. Everything is better in moderation.

The financial burden of pain

Besides the inconvenience it can cause on an individual level, pain can be a huge financial burden for society. According to various studies commissioned by the Canadian Pain Society, 15 to 29 percent of Canadians suffer from chronic pain, and its prevalence increases with age.[4] In Canada, estimates place chronic-pain-related health-care costs at around $6 billion per year and lost productivity costs at some $37 billion per year.[5]

The statistics speak for themselves. According to a study by the Centers for Disease Control and Prevention, in 2016, 20 percent of adults in the United States had chronic pain, with 8 percent experiencing "high-impact chronic pain"—pain so severe that it frequently limits their life activities or work. Studies in Canada have found similar figures, with higher numbers of women afflicted by chronic pain.[6] If we apply these percentages to today's demographics, this means that more than fifty million Americans and eight million Canadians suffer from chronic pain. What's more, the incidence of chronic pain and illness is expected to continue rising over the next decades due to an aging population.[7]

According to a National Population Health Survey conducted by Statistics Canada, individuals with severe chronic pain sought medical advice more often (on average, 12.9 versus 3.8 visits to the doctor's office) and were hospitalized for longer than other individuals (3.9 versus 0.7 days of hospitalization).[8]

Health economists at Johns Hopkins University writing in *The Journal of Pain* reported in 2012 that the cost of chronic pain in the United States is as high as $635 billion a year, which is more than the yearly costs of cancer ($243 billion), heart disease ($309 billion), or diabetes ($188 billion).[9] These figures take into account health-care costs as well as the drop in productivity attributable to chronic pain.

As we can see, the problem of pain is swallowing up enormous amounts of money. The cost of treating pain, coupled with related disabilities, is crippling our society. Clearly, something needs to be done, not only to bring these costs under control, but first and foremost to restore a decent quality of life to those who are suffering.

How pain affects our quality of life

Individuals suffering from chronic pain pay a heavy price on every level. Chronic pain is a burden not only for the sufferers themselves but also for the people around them. It diminishes their quality of life and stifles their creativity. Physical pain increases mortality and the incidence of illness in general, but particularly among the elderly. Pain constantly stimulates the sympathetic nervous system, which regulates heart rate and countless other functions in the body, and the resulting stress can lead to a significant hormonal imbalance. Pain can therefore be a trigger for many complex and chronic illnesses as well as a symptom of a preexisting condition.

Because pain goes hand in hand with anger, frustration, and desperation, physical suffering rarely exists without psychological suffering. Anxiety and sleep disorders are just some of the ripple effects that can further taint an already-diminished quality of life. Even more serious are depression, social withdrawal, and suicidal thoughts, the risks of which are only too real for people who don't understand their pain or are desperately searching for a solution.

ULTIMATELY, PAIN IS a problem we should never ignore. In the pages that follow, we'll explore the meaning of pain and its many causes, as well as the actions we can take to remedy, alleviate, or at least live better with it.

CHAPTER 2

The Meaning of Pain

||||||||||||||||||||||||||||||||||||||||||||||||||||||||||||

Pain is the doorway to the here and now.

DAVID WHYTE

O VER THE YEARS, I've spent a lot of time thinking about the question of suffering in the world. I'm sure most doctors would say that relieving their patients' pain is important to them, but I think that I've pursued this goal with a particular focus, given that I've always looked at human beings in three dimensions: physical, psychological, and spiritual.

Existential questions have always intrigued me, and my many forays into various metaphysical fields have done little to quench my thirst for greater knowledge. Before I went to medical school, I found myself at a series of forks in the road and was unsure which way to turn. After high school I went to a college that was run by Sulpician monks, and for a while I felt drawn to the priesthood, until my raging adolescent hormones took the upper hand and I became infatuated with the opposite sex. Then I was torn between pursuing medicine and going into field biology—I was just as passionate about animals and nature as I was about human beings. I eventually made up my mind when I asked a friend who was a priest and a biology professor which path I should follow. After subjecting me to a career-orientation questionnaire, he handed down a clear recommendation, telling me that no matter how much I loved animals, my vocation was to help people.

I've always felt like a therapist at heart, in the sense that a therapist's primary duty is to serve the patient. Medicine may well be grounded in science, but above all else it is an art, since the human body will never be a machine we can simply service. We don't treat pain; we treat *people* who are in pain. The best kind of doctor is the kind who treats the patient and not the illness.

Pain and suffering are complex things to explain. Over the next pages, we'll examine them through a broad, scientific lens—without losing sight of the philosophical and spiritual aspects, since we are all three-dimensional beings. We know that as human beings, we are more than a physical body. We have an emotional body too, something that exists within us and permeates our entire physical being. It's through these two bodies that we experience either pain or suffering, or both.

How pain makes us suffer

If there's one thing I've learned from all my years of treating chronic pain, it's that a sense of well-being can make all the difference in how we experience pain. But, you might ask, how can psychological well-being exist when pain is eating away at us? Can we feel pain and still be happy and satisfied in our lives?

In other words, can we be in pain without suffering? Can pain even exist without suffering? And how is pain different from suffering?

As we saw in Chapter 1, the experience of pain can vary tremendously depending on the situation and the person. Our emotions, which are subjective by their very nature, color our feelings of pain and can transpose them into a higher register. Thus pain often turns into suffering, even though they're not the same thing. Pain is an uncomfortable physical sensation—an unpleasant feeling, but not one tinged with fear. Suffering, however, is unique to humans, because we convert pain to suffering in our minds. Pain tends to get worse when we become aware of it: once our feelings of fear, anticipation, and desperation come into play, another, even more intense wave of pain washes over us.

You might walk into the corner of a table and feel pain in your leg—nothing more, nothing less. Or that pain might prompt the realization that your physical mobility is decreasing due to your recent heart attack and your diabetes, triggering despair and turning the pain into suffering.

Many a time, I've seen patients who were suffering terribly after an operation. I listened to what they told me and questioned them about the nature and intensity of their pain. Very often, I could tell they were fearful and apprehensive about what was going to happen to them. This new pain, they thought, was going to be life-changing. Typically, they felt a lot of concern and resentment about entering a new phase in their lives, which they imagined would be bleak and devoid of all hope of recovery. However, when I explained more about their illness, the positive changes that the surgery might bring about, and the quality of life they stood to gain, the difference it made was astounding. Their suffering appeared to melt away as they realized that even with some residual pain, they could begin to function normally again. They needed to understand the real effects of their pain and break free of the fear that was making them suffer so much.

One thing is clear: we have to rid ourselves of our apprehension, judgment, and fear around pain—otherwise we risk being drawn into suffering as a way of life.

A lesson from Buddhism

Beyond the questions it raises for individuals, suffering has been a topic of religious and philosophical reflection throughout history and across civilizations. One approach that can teach us a lot about suffering and the different ways to manage it is Buddhism.

Twenty-five hundred years ago, there was a young prince, Siddhārtha Gautama, who lived in an opulent palace. His father, the king, built a wall around the whole palace to make sure his son never learned that misery existed on earth. Young Siddhārtha only knew the beauty around him, since he never left the palace grounds. Until one day, when his curiosity got the better of him and he went to see what lay beyond the walls. To his great surprise, he saw not only beauty and joy in the outside world, but also misery, sickness, and death.

When he was twenty-nine years old, Siddhārtha decided to relinquish his princely existence and become a wandering monk, begging for food in order to survive. He wanted to try to understand the origin of suffering and find ways to overcome it. And so, he followed the teachings of the spiritual masters, but he was not always satisfied with the answers he found.

Since the masters had taught him that the body and its desires were obstacles to spiritual growth, he subjected himself to great hardship and suffering.

As he neared the end of his life, he heard a musician playing a lute. At that moment, he realized that if the strings of the instrument were too loose, they would not make any sound, but if they were too taut, they would break. Only when the strings were subjected to the right amount of tension would they produce a pleasant sound. He learned that the way forward was to find the right balance, and so he no longer forced such hardship on himself.

Determined more than ever to find the answers to his questions, he sat down beneath the Bodhi tree and immersed himself in profound meditation, resolving to get up again only once he had found truth. Several days later, by the light of the full moon, he attained enlightenment and finally understood the cycle of birth, life, and death. From that moment on, he became known as the Buddha (the enlightened one; a knower). He was thirty-five years old, and he devoted the rest of his life to disseminating his teachings on compassion.

THE FOUR NOBLE TRUTHS: AN INSIGHT FOR MEDICINE

In Buddhism, the Four Noble Truths represent the Buddha's first sermon after attaining spiritual enlightenment beneath the Bodhi tree. The first Noble Truth is expressed by the word *dukkha*, which, depending on the interpretation, means "all is suffering," "precariousness," or "dissatisfaction." *Dukkha* stresses the importance of suffering to the human condition. We'll all experience suffering, sooner or later: birth is suffering, death is suffering, and between the two lies more suffering, be it mental or physical. Sickness, aging, the loss of a companion, change—anything we feel or perceive may become suffering. This may seem pessimistic, but it's simply the acceptance that suffering is a certainty in life. In fact, the Buddha's message is optimistic, as according to him, we can rise above dissatisfaction and suffering by heeding the Four Noble Truths.

The second Noble Truth addresses the origin of suffering, because if we want to eliminate suffering, we must know its causes.

The third Noble Truth concerns the end of suffering. Once we know its origin, it will be easier for us to work to free ourselves from it and achieve final liberation, as the Buddha puts it.

The fourth Noble Truth shows us the path to the end of suffering, through a set of principles called the Eightfold Path. It's also known as the Middle Way, because it avoids extremes in the search for happiness.

It's interesting to compare these Four Noble Truths to the therapeutic process doctors follow with their patients. First, the doctor assesses the patient's symptoms. Second, the doctor diagnoses the patient's illness or suffering and seeks the cause. Third, the doctor finds a remedy and method for healing the patient. Fourth, the doctor encourages the patient to adopt a lifestyle change and develop sustainable healthier habits. This is the path any good practitioner should follow with a patient, and it was established more than 2,500 years ago. It's also the approach I'll discuss in this book.

A road we must travel, and a road to nowhere

As human beings, we're always making discoveries, and pain is one path of our evolution. Children learn through pain—every time they burn their hand, pinch a finger, scrape their knee, sip a drink that's too hot, or insult a friend and get a punch on the nose in return. Every painful experience delivers new teachings in the school of life.

In our world, friction is what seems to make everything function. Newton's laws of motion tell us that friction is a force that works in opposition when one body moves over another. This force can make a stationary object accelerate. Whether we're talking about electricity, gravitation, or even an accelerating vehicle, it takes friction to make it work. A car can't gain traction if there's no friction beneath its tires; on an icy or oily surface, its wheels will simply spin. According to an old saying, comfort is the graveyard of the soul. In other words, too much ease and well-being in our lives is likely to hold us back or lead to stagnation.

I believe that any illness or pain that suddenly appears doesn't happen by chance. Sickness has a role to play in our lives. If I get the flu, for example, I can deduce that it's because I'm tired, because my immune system needs a boost, or because I hugged so-and-so when I wished them a happy birthday. But that would be looking at my illness on only the surface level.

After all, illness is not a purely biological phenomenon, even if its physical symptoms seem to suggest it. There are many other factors that can affect our immune system, and some of these are psychological. If we explore the hows and whys, we might uncover mismanaged emotions or imbalances in our life that are affecting our energy. The flu will take hold wherever it can flourish. As Louis Pasteur so wisely said, "The germ is nothing, the terrain is everything."

Still, most of us would rather blame an infectious disease on another person or on circumstance, perhaps because we can't grasp that the reason for our illness might lie partly within ourselves. The flu forces me to ask myself some questions. Am I spreading myself too thinly? Or working too hard? What is the flu trying to get me to do or to understand? Perhaps it's trying to tell me to give myself a break? It might force me to rest up for a while, which wouldn't be a bad thing, right? Really, the flu isn't that big a deal when you have the resources to fight it off. And maybe all those secretions coughed up from the lungs and blown out of the nose are the body's way of cleaning itself out?

In my first year of medical school I was working nonstop and caught the mother of all flus: the classic influenza virus, complete with high fever, crippling fatigue, and muscle aches and pains that were so bad even the pressure of the mattress beneath my body felt painful. Bedridden for days, I had to miss all my classes and felt a certain sense of shame about it. But in the months that followed, it felt like I'd turned over a new leaf. Being sick had forced me to develop some new habits that were good for me. I was going to bed earlier and paying attention to my sleep cycles, and I realized that my habits before had made me vulnerable. Once I had recovered, more than ever before I could appreciate the health I had always taken for granted. It struck me how important prevention was, too. From that point on, I felt immensely grateful to be healthy again.

Now, this is not a matter of judgment or of blaming ourselves. It's simply about realizing that sickness and pain can be good teachers, even if they're uninvited. Pain and sickness sometimes have lessons for us, and they're often rooted in psychological distress. I'm convinced that many illnesses arise out of the need to correct an imbalance. Far from being a punishment, they're intended to help us build strength. In most cases, this won't be a pleasant process, but it may bring about a change that will lead to greater harmony in our lives and help us to be more mindful, compassionate, and mature human beings. I believe this is true of much of the pain that we'll need to face and understand over the course of our lives.

The duty of empathy

One of the best remedies for our pain or suffering is another person's empathy. Nowhere is this more true than in the doctor-patient relationship. An attentive, well-intentioned listening ear is the first step in any effective treatment, if not the treatment in itself.

When I was doing my residency, I was keen to learn everything I could about the pathologies of the articular and muscular systems, especially the various forms of arthritis that affect so many people today. I saw so many powerless, helpless patients who were begging for treatment and medication in the hope of finding relief. I remember one rheumatology professor, a tall, stocky, ruddy-cheeked man who spent his time hunched over his desk and used to see patient after patient without getting up. He might have been built like a bear, but his eyes were reduced to tiny specks behind the thick lenses of his magnifying-glass-like spectacles. Was it the glasses that prevented him from seeing the frail lady shuffling over to him with her cane? He didn't even look at her. The only thing he did look at was the hefty stack of papers in this elderly patient's file. Still without looking up at her or even saying hello, he started quizzing her about the medication she was on. I was standing off to the side of his desk, observing the visit in silence.

The patient's answers were somewhat unclear, since she barely had time to finish a sentence before the rheumatologist fired off another question. Three questions in, I was flabbergasted that he still hadn't looked at her. The visit lasted barely five minutes, and the poor patient left his office the same way she had come in, without once making eye contact with the doctor who had written her a prescription. All his other patients came and went the exact same way. The doctor spent very little time listening to them, next to no time examining them, and not one second showing the slightest compassion for any of these people suffering from arthritis. It would have done them so much good if he'd simply given them a smile and said hello, and if he'd taken the time to listen to them or empathize with them the way many doctors do. I was still a student, but in spite of my youth and lack of experience, I knew that what I had seen that afternoon was not the kind of medicine I would ever practice. From that point, whenever any of my patients needed a referral to a rheumatologist, I always sent them to colleagues whom I knew had the patience and empathy to help people with these types of conditions.

One day, a patient of mine decided to consult a rheumatologist who was not one I usually recommended. I was happy to hear that she had finally found someone who was able to relieve her pain, since she had already consulted several specialists and her particular case of arthritis was very complex. She told me how the doctor practically fell over himself to shake her hand as soon as she walked into his office, listened to what she said very attentively, and looked at her with compassion. Finally, she had found the specialist for her! She went on to describe the doctor: a tall and stocky elderly man who suffered from arthritis himself.

As chance would have it, it was the very same rheumatologist I mentioned earlier. Clearly, his own condition and experience of pain had softened his bedside manner and made him an empathetic doctor who could finally show compassion for his patients. I dare say it had made him more human—a great example of how sickness can bring positive change.

I didn't want to spoil my patient's good mood, so I told her that her new specialist was the professor who had taught me the most when I was studying rheumatology! It wasn't far from the truth, in fact, because so many years previously, my experience with that specialist had taught me precisely the kind of doctor I didn't want to become. But most important was that this specialist eventually found his way and became a compassionate therapist who was able to bring relief and reassurance to his patients.

The power to change

In a way, it's not surprising that we suffer, because we don't have the power to control our physical and emotional bodies, nor do we sufficiently understand them. What's more, sometimes we behave in harmful ways—not intentionally, but because we don't know better. Everything we do in our lives tends to echo back at us. We've created the society we live in, and that society is suffering more and more. Even without our realizing it, the environment we live in can influence us; it can have positive or harmful effects on our psyche and change our physical reality.

If we want to change the course of our existence, it's important to think about what's going on in our lives and reflect on why the things that happen to us happen. I've always believed that we alone are responsible for what we do with our lives. Let's act now to build a different future. Let's be mindful about what life brings our way and ask ourselves *why* things happen, because it isn't by chance. Let's be mindful of *who* we are and the qualities we have to share as well as the imperfections we'd like to change.

We tend to hang on to old habits and stick to what we know because it's familiar, even though it makes our lives ever more complicated. It seems to me that it's often easier to muddle our way through a familiar discomfort than to overcome the insecurity that change can bring, even if we stand to reap the benefits in the long run. Let's shed the skins we no longer need and rid ourselves of old habits that only stand in our way or cause us pain. It's time to make way for a better life and a promising future. If we do, the path of suffering might well fall into disuse.

I'm reminded of the movie *Groundhog Day*, starring Bill Murray—a film that's well worth a rewatch. The frivolous-sounding title belies a story with a powerful message about the repetitive nature of our habits: when we go around in circles, we leave no room for positive change in our lives. This movie has inspired much philosophical discussion and given many people a wake-up call about self-perpetuating situations in their lives. When Murray's character, Phil, realizes that he's living the same day over and over again, initially he goes along with the scenario—until he finally gets too annoyed with constantly reliving the same torment. He ends up making the most of the situation and changing the routine that he was so used to, but that brought nothing positive to his life. Ultimately, it's desperation, irritation, and suffering that spur him to draw on his experiences and help himself and others to break free.

Reliving the same negativity day after day ends up taking its toll on us in real life, too. Irritation, discomfort, and suffering are often what push us to break the cycle. I would argue that for many of us, sheer exasperation with pain is the real driver of change.

                           ‖‖‖‖‖‖‖‖‖‖‖‖‖‖‖‖‖‖‖‖‖‖‖‖‖

BEFORE WE CAN pinpoint the changes we need to make to control or eradicate our pain, we need to understand where it's coming from. In the next chapter, we'll put our finger on the possible sources of pain and look at some of its physical and psychological causes.

CHAPTER 3

Why Am I in Pain?

||||||||||||||||||||||||||||||||||||||||||||||||||||||||||||||||||

When you are suffering, confront the pain:
it will comfort you and teach you something.
ALEXANDRE DUMAS

B EFORE WE CAN treat—and in an ideal world, eradicate—chronic
pain, it goes without saying that we must first understand its origin. Am I in pain because the lifestyle I've been living for years
has been causing inflammation? Or am I in pain because I'm overus-
ing my muscles, tendons, or ligaments, or because I injured myself
and it hasn't healed yet? In this chapter we'll look at the mechanical,
physical, and environmental causes of pain. We'll also run through
the psychological factors that can be sources of pain.

Biological and environmental causes of pain
||||||||||||||||||||||||||||||||||||||||||||||||||||||||||

Generally speaking, physical musculoskeletal pain can be attributed
to two main causes: inflammation (acute or chronic) or the persistent
stretching of ligaments or tendons.

ACUTE VS. CHRONIC INFLAMMATION

Acute inflammation is a defense mechanism. It's the body's natural reaction to fight off an attack from the inside or outside, which might be from bacteria, a virus, bruising, or inflammatory molecules. When the body experiences a trauma caused by a cut, blow, or shock, its immediate response is to trigger pain, heat, redness, and swelling—the four corners of acute pain. At the same time, it sets off a series of chemical reactions to repair the injury to the tissue, and the inflammation tends to subside in a matter of weeks. Acute inflammation isn't a bad thing, therefore; it's a survival mechanism. Think of it as the body's way of sounding the alarm. However, this mechanism can work against us and become the cause of many pains and ailments if it becomes chronic.

When acute inflammation fails to repair the damage and persists for months, a vicious cycle of cellular degradation begins, producing harmful inflammatory substances within the body. We refer to this abnormal phase as **chronic inflammation**. Because of the constant influx of toxic cells, the tissue is unable to rebuild itself. If the injury does heal, it will typically lead to **fibrosis**—a thickening and scarring of tissue that can hinder the functioning of that part of the body.

You probably won't notice the symptoms of chronic inflammation in the beginning, because they tend to sneak up on you. It often begins with common and varying ailments, such as a sinus infection, muscle or joint pain, digestive or dermatological issues, a lack of feeling, loss of balance, or even the dreaded chronic fatigue.

THE CAUSES OF CHRONIC INFLAMMATION

Today we recognize chronic inflammation as a response to changes in the body caused by our environment, poor diet, sedentariness, pollution, or digestive system disruptions. Chronic inflammation produces toxic free radicals and causes oxidative stress, which is a little like rust spreading through the body and seizing the inner workings. Because inflammation is conducive to tissue degeneration, it can lead to premature aging in many ways. For instance, a hardening and obstruction of the arteries can result in heart disease and increase the risk of stroke. Other examples include diabetes, osteoarthritis, and degenerative illnesses such as Alzheimer's disease. We can also point the finger at chronic inflammation for any number of "itises" that are increasingly plaguing the modern world—think arthritis, vasculitis, and many other autoimmune diseases.

Many roads can lead to chronic inflammation, whether it's too much sugar or too much insulin, too high a proportion of omega-6 to omega-3 fatty acids, abdominal obesity, pervasive stress, insomnia, toxins in the environment or on our plates, GMOs, allergy-inducing additives, or a decline in sex hormones that interferes with our normal functioning. Rogue inflammation can silently seep its way into the body through many doors, including the mouth (gingivitis) and the gut (harmful bacteria). What's more, any kind of food intolerance can disrupt intestinal-wall function.

In today's advanced medical practice, doctors are increasingly inclined to screen for factors that indicate inflammation when they prescribe blood work for patients. Tests are now available to measure CRP (C-reactive protein), fibrinogen, ESR (erythrocyte sedimentation rate), TNF alpha, and interleukins, for instance.

Sedentariness is also becoming a major cause of chronic inflammation,[1] because many of us aren't as physically active as we should be, and our circulatory systems lose the ability to eliminate all the harmful inflammatory molecules we encounter. It's also important to make sure we get enough rest and regular sleep. In the next chapter, we'll look at some of the things that can help, such as omega-3 fatty acids, gamma-linolenic acid (GLA), *Boswellia serrata*, collagen, and turmeric.

As a conference speaker, I often talk about how chronic inflammation can be a silent killer. Many of us have no idea just how much our way of life in the last fifty or so years has become disconnected from nature, upsetting our biochemical balance. The good news is that we can correct these inflammatory problems by changing our lifestyle, as we'll see later.

ANTI-INFLAMMATORY DRUGS:
A REAL SOLUTION?

You might be wondering whether you can just take anti-inflammatory drugs every day to get rid of chronic inflammation. This might seem logical, but don't count on it to solve the problem. Anti-inflammatory drugs can have many harmful side effects. Vioxx, for example, has destroyed the lives of hundreds of thousands of people by causing increased risk of myocardial infarction, stroke, and sudden death. Studies on the biochemical function of anti-inflammatory drugs have shown that they lead to vascular damage.[2] The same goes for other COX-2 inhibitors (drugs like Celebrex), which may also end up being pulled from the market given the similarities in their composition to Vioxx.

According to scientific data released in 2017, all anti-inflammatory drugs can lead not only to gastric problems and high blood pressure but also to a range of cardiological and cerebrovascular diseases. That's right—even over-the-counter drugs like ibuprofen can increase the risk of vascular disease.[3] Blood pressure was shown to increase in a significant proportion of individuals who were taking anti-inflammatories. We would be wise to use all non-steroidal anti-inflammatory drugs (NSAIDS) with caution, in small doses, and for short periods.

GUT PROBLEMS AND CHRONIC INFLAMMATION

You know how we say we have a gut feeling about something? Well, it turns out there's a good reason for that saying. Experts are increasingly observing connections between intestinal disorders and a number of illnesses. Together with a healthy intestinal barrier, gut flora and bacteria are essential to our overall health. We know today that an imbalance in the gut affects the body's capacity to manage pain, stress, depression, chronic illness, and cellular immunity.[4]

We also know that people with a so-called irritable bowel, who can experience bloating, gas, and alternating diarrhea and constipation, tend to be more prone to pain, depression, and stress.[5] Unfortunately, doctors continue to dismiss many patients as hypochondriacs despite it being increasingly acknowledged that inadequate intestinal flora, rogue bacteria, and food intolerances can create chronic inflammation in the intestinal mucosa. These factors may ultimately lead to the development of micro-ulcers in the intestinal wall—referred to as intestinal permeability or leaky gut syndrome—leaving the door open for more inflammation, pain, and chronic illness to creep in.[6] While some doctors remain skeptical about leaky gut syndrome, it is a real condition, as studies have increasingly shown. We'll go into this in more detail in Chapter 4.

I've often encountered patients who were suffering from chronic headaches that disappeared when they switched to a more suitable diet. When our gut is sick, we're often not aware of it. But more and more research is connecting the dots between our mood and the quality of our gut bacteria, and revealing how an unhealthy gut can lead to insufficient levels of mood-regulating neurotransmitters.[7]

WHAT ARE NEUROTRANSMITTERS?

Neurotransmitters are the body's chemical messengers, made up essentially of amino acids. **Neuro** stands for neurons—nerve cells—and they're called **transmitters** because they transmit and relay messages. A little like hormones, these molecules influence all our bodily functions. The brain and gut contain a large quantity of neurotransmitters that are crucial to our well-being. So far researchers have identified more than a hundred types of neurotransmitters. The main neurotransmitters, and the functions and feelings they are associated with, include **serotonin** (happiness), **dopamine** (mood and motivation), GABA (gamma-aminobutyric acid, a sedative), **melatonin** (sleep and wakefulness), **glutamate** (excitement), **acetylcholine** (muscle activity), and **epinephrine** (alertness).

THE FORGOTTEN LIGAMENTS

While inflammation is the number one cause of pain, the number two cause is one we still know very little about: damage to our ligaments and tendons. Microtearing and stretching of these structures can persist until the underlying cause is resolved, and when they're chronically stretched and distended, they can send pain signals to our brain even if the inflammation has gone away. This is why doctors no longer prescribe anti-inflammatory drugs as a long-term solution for chronic pain caused by damaged ligaments or tendons.

To help explain the mechanism behind many of the aches and pains we feel in our back and other parts of our body, let's talk for a moment about ligaments. The role they play tends to be underappreciated—some might say they're the ugly ducklings of medicine.

Ligaments are dense, whitish structures of connective tissue, mostly made of collagen, that hold our bones together and stabilize our joints. They're relatively short—like small, tightly woven ropes—and very strong. However, they're not very elastic, they receive very little blood flow, and they take longer to repair than tendons and muscles. When a ligament is damaged, it makes our joints more mobile and forces them to work too hard—a bit like how a loose steering column on a car can cause the tires to wear prematurely. This in turn leads to greater stress on the tendons and muscles, which may enter an inflammatory phase as a result.

Back in the 1980s, the medical world was full of talk about muscles and joints, but very little was being said about ligaments as a source of chronic pain. That was when I first encountered the great British orthopedic physician Dr. James Cyriax, who developed the notion of **ligamentary pain**—the referred pain caused by a faulty ligament.

LIGAMENTS VS. TENDONS

Tendons connect both extremities of a muscle to the bone and enable movement. They're small, white connectors that attach to the muscle where it narrows. **Ligaments** are short, tough, whitish particles that attach one bone to another. Ligaments don't contract the way muscles do. Think of them as tiny threads that hold our skeleton together whether we're moving or at rest.

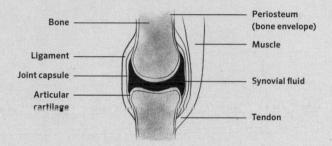

Ligaments tend to have a weak point where they connect to the bone. Many ligament injuries start here, in what's called the **periosteum**—the envelope that covers the bone, where tearing tends to occur.

In fact, long before Dr. Cyriax, in a book published in the 1950s, the American neurosurgeon Dr. George Hackett suggested that ligaments were responsible for a high proportion of referred pain.[8] This realization—that a dorsal or lumbar ligament in the spine could cause pain up to three feet away—opened up whole new avenues for treating issues at their source. Dr. Hackett even mapped out the various channels in the body that could carry referred pain.

In the following diagram, based on Dr. Hackett's map, we can see the sacroiliac (SI) ligaments in the pelvis and the areas of the buttocks, legs, and even the feet, where pain can radiate. Sometimes, the area where the pain originates will not feel painful, and the pain will only manifest in a distant area—and this pain can't be explained by a nerve path. That's why, if you feel pain radiating into your leg, you shouldn't jump to the conclusion that it's a herniated disc, requiring surgery. The observations Dr. Hackett made, however, are generally absent from medical textbooks.[9]

Dr. Hackett's ligament map

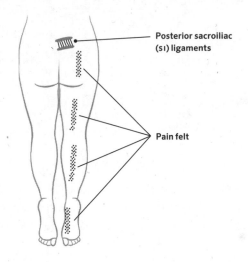

Posterior sacroiliac (si) ligaments

Pain felt

It's important to locate the origin of any referred pain so we can treat it at the source. Interestingly, doctors can check for referred pain by injecting a minute quantity of xylocaine—an anesthetic—into an injured, torn, or painful ligament in the lumbar region. Any referred pain in the buttock and leg will disappear in minutes, and the origin point of the pain will be clear.

Ligaments can create their fair share of back and leg pain, as well as sciatica (inflammation along the sciatic nerve). The **sacroiliac (si) ligaments**, voluminous structures that attach the sacrum (the large, triangular bone at the base of the spine) to the iliac bone (the "wings" of the pelvis), can play a debilitating role when it comes to back problems. They're often subjected to a lot of stress and micro-movements at the sacroiliac joint, which can cause lumbar pain.

We might assume the pelvis is a stable part of the body that doesn't have moving joints. The role ligaments play in the ankle is perhaps clearer to see, since there are so many of these little structures supporting the joint. Most of the time, ligaments are to blame when we twist our ankle. When they're stretched, it results in pain and swelling. In severe cases, one or more ligaments may even be torn.[10]

Ligaments in the ankle susceptible to a sprain

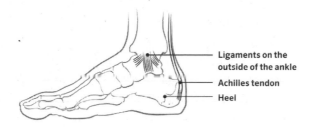

Ligaments on the outside of the ankle

Achilles tendon

Heel

WHEN ACUTE BECOMES CHRONIC

For many years, I've treated patients whose pain could no longer be relieved by anti-inflammatories or analgesics (painkillers). All they wanted was to regain a decent quality of life, and conventional medicine was powerless to help. Many people with injuries continue to suffer terribly with no hope of relief after exhausting all the recognized forms of therapy available. In the case of many of these painful situations, the inflammation has essentially subsided, yet the pain persists because of malfunctions in the ligament structures. When the tiny nerves in torn ligaments are damaged, they keep sending pain signals until the structures are repaired. All ligaments are made up of these sensitive fibers. If the ligament is subjected to constant and abnormal tension, these sensitive nerve fibers trigger painful stimuli.

Instability in the ligaments can also cause exaggerated movement in the joints and other muscle and tendon structures, which may lead to further problems—loss of cartilage, meniscus tears, and contractures in other muscles—all of which generate even more pain. A manual examination with thorough palpating of the area can reveal all these damaged nerve, ligament, and tendon structures.

This is why hands-off treatments that are limited to prescribing anti-inflammatories over and over lead to mixed or short-lived results, and may even be harmful. We'll revisit treatment options in Chapter 6.

COLLAGEN PROBLEMS

Whatever the source of the injury, it's important not only to treat the inflammation, but also to repair the broken connective tissue— ligaments as well as collagen. When collagen is damaged and not replaced, the ligament stretches abnormally and remains a source of unresolved pain.[11] Leading a healthy way of life, doing personalized rehabilitation exercises, taking dietary supplements, and having targeted injections in the affected area can all help to partially rebuild these damaged structures.

WHAT IS COLLAGEN?

You'll hear a lot of talk about **collagen** in the beauty world—think face-lifts and fuller lips—but there's much more to this molecule. Collagen is a protein that forms thin fibers to create a safety net of sorts between cells. It makes tissue more resistant to stretching and can be found mainly in ligaments, tendons, joint capsules (broad, ligament-like membranes that contain lubricating synovial fluid), and skin. Collagen is actually the most abundant protein in the body, but it declines rapidly in quantity with age and inactivity. Together with **elastin**, it provides strength and elasticity. Collagen plays a role in healing, because it forms wherever tissue has been cut or pulled; the origin of the word can be traced back to the Greek *kólla*, meaning glue. And if collagen is mixed with water, it becomes gelatin, the sticky substance used in many foods and beauty products.

Collagen problems frequently occur following a fall or a vehicle or workplace accident, and they can also be caused by aging. Sometimes the gravity-induced damage that comes with age is only too visible, much to the satisfaction of beauty clinics everywhere.

One of the ailments associated with a lack of collagen is scurvy. This disease is caused by a deficiency of vitamin C—which plays a role in the formation of collagen—and affects connective tissue everywhere in the body, including the blood vessels. Indigenous people in North America were no strangers to scurvy. In 1535, during Jacques Cartier's second voyage of discovery to Canada, twenty-five men in his crew succumbed to the disease. Cartier noticed that Domagaya, the son of an Iroquois chief with whom he had returned to France after his first journey, had also contracted scurvy. When he saw Domagaya again several months later, he was the picture of good health. Cartier asked him the secret of his recovery, and learned that making a tea from the needles and bark of the eastern white cedar tree, common to the area, was a natural remedy. Nowadays, a powerful antioxidant called pycnogenol is extracted from the bark of these trees—proof that the Iroquois knew what they were doing!

POOR POSTURE

Even before computers became commonplace, poor posture was to blame for a great many ailments, particularly back pain caused by sitting without adequate back support. However, the advent of computer-based work has created a veritable epidemic of musculoskeletal problems. These can range from sore spots between the shoulder blades, caused by sitting for too long in a hunched position, to bursitis (nerve compression) and carpal tunnel syndrome in the shoulder and wrist, caused by the repetitive movements of using a mouse. And neck pain is one of the most frequent consequences of sitting at a computer workstation. When we spend long hours in front of a screen, there is constant muscle tension in our neck and shoulders.

In adults, computer work is so widespread it can be a real headache or a pain in the neck (literally!). Many of us tend to lean forward for a better view of what's on our screen. This head-forward position creates muscle tension in the anterior and posterior triangle of the neck, which can frequently lead to a headache or sore neck. Proper posture can help us avoid these kinds of problems.[12]

Correct...
Our head, shoulders, and arms must all be in an ergonomic position when working at a computer. Tension in the shoulders is a common symptom of our hands tapping away at the keyboard without proper support. At the same time, sitting in the same position puts stress on the entire muscle mass of the back of the neck, shoulders, and arms, which can send pain down between the shoulder blades. This can also overload the trapezius, the diamond-shaped muscle connecting the back of the head (occiput), the shoulder blades, and the lower dorsal region.

Relax...
Our eye muscles work pretty hard too when they're staring at a screen all day. When we're at a computer, our eyes tend to focus on one point (the screen) rather than looking at things around us both near and far away. Staring at one stationary spot can cause eye strain and headaches.

Remaining in a stationary position also causes muscle fatigue. Inactivity slows our circulation and hardens our muscles, and tension and fatigue soon set in. If your work requires you to spend a long time at a computer, it's a good idea to take your eyes off the screen and look around the room every twenty minutes or so. Look up, down, and to either side, or draw a circle in the air with your finger and follow it with your eyes, first close to your face and then farther away. Rotate your shoulders. Stand up and stretch your spine. Tuck your chin and rotate your neck from side to side (see Chapter 5 for a little inspiration). Then you can get back to work. The idea is to shake off the tension before any signs of pain appear. Otherwise, a vicious cycle can set in: tension creates pain, pain in turn creates more tension, and before you know it, you could find yourself battling a chronic pain in the neck.

Breathe!

It's so important to relax, and one way to do that is by using deep-breathing techniques. At regular intervals, take three very deep breaths. You should feel your collarbones move up and down and your chest and belly fill with air and empty again.

HORMONAL CHANGES

One of the most familiar and striking examples of change in hormonal balance is menopause. Menopause is caused by decreasing levels of sex hormones—not just estrogen and progesterone, but also testosterone, which women secrete too, albeit in lower concentrations than men. Menopause is often the trigger for psychological and mood disorders, as well as all manner of ailments: poor sleep, joint pain, tension in the neck, headaches, pain during sex due to dryness in the mucous membranes, not to mention the risk of osteoporosis.

Helen, age fifty-nine, had been suffering intense headaches almost daily for over ten years. She had consulted several doctors, including some specialists, and had undergone a number of tests, but the results had always come back negative. She had tried various medications without success and even had to quit her job because her headaches were so pervasive. She had also tried alternative approaches—chiropractors, physiotherapists, osteopaths, and naturopaths—all in vain. When she consulted with me, she told me her headaches had started at the same time as her menopause.

Other than the headaches, she showed very few other negative effects of menopause.

She had mentioned the connection between her headaches and the onset of her menopause to all the health professionals she saw, but none of them had showed any interest. She drove for hours to come and see me, determined to get to the bottom of her problem and make sure I took the hormonal process into consideration. In my opinion, it was certainly a plausible theory. Since she had no contraindication to hormone replacement therapy, I prescribed her bioidentical hormones with estrogen and progesterone. Three months later, she called me to tell me her headaches had finally disappeared.

Pain and our emotions

Even if it's the physical body that's suffering, the ultimate source of many of our ailments lies first and foremost in our psyche. Only recently have we begun to recognize the significance of our emotions in generating pain and chronic illness. Welcome to the world of psychosomatics.[13]

As human beings, our body and mind are intertwined, so it's only natural for there to be a mental dimension to our various ailments. Have you ever noticed how when you hear some bad news, whether it turns out to be true or not, your heart suddenly starts pounding, your pulse begins to race, you feel a headache coming on, or your stomach feels like it's tying itself in knots? We might wish for a miracle pill to rid ourselves of all that ails us, but unfortunately, there's no such magic solution. Instead, we must look backward and sometimes dig deep into our past to figure out what sent our psyche out of whack. We might discover that our ailments are rooted in emotional events in our past that may still be troubling us. Simply being aware of these issues—"emotional knots," we might call them—can help us to untangle chronic pain, sometimes surprisingly quickly.

TOXIC EMOTIONS AND STRESS

Just as the food we eat affects our bodies, the "psychological food" that our minds take in can cause us illness and suffering if it is toxic. It's increasingly recognized that negative feelings and emotional states, such as anger, sadness, anxiety, and depression, have pathological effects, and that our immune defenses and hormonal balance end up paying the price.[14] Our thoughts trigger emotions, and these emotions affect our nervous and endocrine systems, which in turn influence our cellular immunity. We call this the **psychoneuro-endocrine response**.

You know how we say someone gets on our nerves? The expression we use in Quebec translates to "you're getting on my spleen." That's no coincidence. The spleen, pancreas, and digestive system are all in the solar plexus area, which is essentially the hub for our sympathetic nervous system and our emotional being. More and more in the modern world, we're living under the yoke of emotional ups and downs, fatigue, and pressure, and losing touch with our body's natural rhythm and cycles. The drive to keep busy and sacrifice ourselves for our work is often the result of unresolved emotional issues. We simply forget that we need to follow a natural cycle of activity and rest. Having an overactive neuroendocrine system puts us at risk of getting sick, which may ultimately be what forces us to slow down. If we don't take the time now to hit the pause button for our health, we'll have to do it down the line and risk being out of action for much longer and with a far greater price to pay.

What's more, psychological stress from our distant past can be hiding in our internal organs. On several occasions I've observed how abdominal pain in adult women whose test results all came back normal was rooted in a painful memory from childhood (such as incest, for example). The problem is often so repressed that the source seems to have disappeared. The tip of the iceberg might be all that is apparent, but the painful symptoms are sustained by what persists beneath the surface—which all weighs heavily on the person's quality of life.[15] A renowned surgeon who teaches at the Université de Sherbrooke,

Dr. Ghislain Devroede, wrote an entire book on the topic of what stomach pain can tell us about our past.[16] He has observed this issue so frequently that in many patients' cases he has called off their surgery and referred them for psychotherapy instead.

In situations like these, psychotherapy and even hypnotherapy can often be very useful in pinpointing the cause of an ailment, as well as in the treatment itself. Contrary to what you might think, I believe it's beneficial for a person to dig up their painful memories, because time alone won't erase the psychosomatic consequences of distressing events we experienced earlier in life. Once we identify this distress, we can treat the cause of the physical symptoms, which might otherwise keep getting worse and potentially degenerate into more serious issues. For many patients, going through this process can finally draw a line under years of endless searching, which is often complex and painful in itself.

In children, digestive issues can sometimes camouflage emotions that are too much for their mind to process, so are unconsciously transferred to their "brain down below." Children are particularly vulnerable to the impact of events in their little lives. Their minds are like cameras that capture anything and everything—sometimes magnified far larger than life!—and a blemish in an otherwise clear-blue sky can eventually manifest in the form of sickness.

THE EMOTIONAL SIDE OF LUMBAR SPRAIN

We've all suffered back pain at some point in our lives. It's such a frequent complaint that we tend to trivialize it, accepting that the slightest wrong move might lead to the dreaded backache. When it happens, we might put the blame on the pencil we dropped on the floor and bent over to pick up. But is that all there is to it? Could the pencil really be the cause of a lumbar sprain that persists for a month or, worse still, a herniated disc that might send the patient to the operating table? Or rather, could it simply be the trigger for a latent issue lurking deep below the surface?[17]

In fact, at the root of many lumbar sprains is stress or an underlying emotional state—perhaps chronic anxiety or suppressed anger.

The muscle acts like a sponge, absorbing the negative emotion and effectively making it a part of the muscle. The prolonged contracture of that muscle then leads to insufficient circulation, and muscle waste, lactic acid, and other substances start to build up. And so the muscle becomes toxic, so to speak, reflecting the toxicity of our emotions, thoughts, and negative beliefs. These toxic emotions can disrupt the contraction of our muscles and create painful spasms in our back.

This is a very common occurrence, but unfortunately we don't always take the time to delve deeply into what's causing our lumbar sprains. Sometimes, however, we're forced to do so when the pain persists, recurs, or gets worse.

One of the many patients I've treated for back pain was able to find some relief through massage and physiotherapy, but his lumbago persisted—until the day when I thought to ask him whether he was happy at work. He then told me how he really didn't get along with his boss. At that point, I was "manipulating" him—applying massage pressure—and as soon as he started talking about his boss, the muscle suddenly became very hard and he complained that the pain was getting worse. And so, I suggested that the conflict with his boss might be to blame for his back pain.

Once he made the connection, he began to practice relaxation techniques and tried to change his attitude toward his superior. He started to see that his unhealthy attitude toward his boss—a man who was well-liked by plenty of other employees—was at the root of his problem. He realized that he himself had been the cause, and that he had held the solution to the problem all along. From that point on, the pain disappeared completely and never returned.

On several occasions, I've seen patients who felt resentment, envy, or jealousy toward their superior. Such negative perceptions often end up turning against the employee themselves as well as their boss. Criticism is a poison that can harm both parties—the person doing the criticizing and the person on the receiving end.

In my opinion, a large proportion of persistent mild back complaints are emotional in origin. Think about the frustration, anger, and aggression we feel from day to day; we try to put it behind us, and in a way we do, literally—right into our backs! When chronic tension becomes too much for our brains to bear, it's as if we channel that tension down into other organs of the body—often the back muscles. And we know that stress is a contractile factor: when we're stressed, we're tight. Could we eventually crack under the pressure of too heavy an emotional burden?

GO EASY ON YOUR LOWER BACK

The lumbar region is the area where the lower vertebrae meet the sacrum. This part of the lower back supports the torso—the entire upper body—so it carries a lot of weight, both physically and metaphorically. The support it provides also has significant psychological and symbolic connotations. Based on many clinical cases, it's become clear to me that this part of the body is essential to our sense of safety. As I spoke with my patients and asked them about their lives at home and at work, it struck me how their psychological tension was related to a situation or event that caused them to feel insecure, which manifested as tightness in the lumbar spine.

I also observed how patients who tended to react strongly to other drivers' lack of courtesy on the road often found their lumbar area tensing up as a reflex when they were driving—so much so that when they got out of the car, the tension they had experienced at the wheel would make them feel stiff and sore. I found that making these patients aware of the situation and encouraging them to relax by doing breathing exercises while driving helped to break their vicious cycle of recurring lower back pain.

Anything that threatens our safety can cause fragility in our lumbar region, which may manifest as lumbar tension, lumbar sprain, or even a herniated disc. I'm talking about safety on every level here, emotional and physical safety included. A threat might stem from trouble in your love life, concerns for the future if your job is on the line, money worries, or even an unsettling political climate. If a patient presents with psychological tension and a chronic compression in the lumbar region, the persistent contracture of the muscle mass will end up affecting the circulation, hydration, and nutrition of the spinal discs. In the long run, the discs can dry out and crack with often the most trivial of actions, resulting in a herniated disc.

It's not surprising that insecurity can have repercussions in our lower back. When we throw our back out, we lose our footing, metaphorically speaking. The pain can be exhausting; our back hunches under the weight of a future that seems uncertain and destabilizing. Insecurity in our back can cripple us from moving forward.

Women tend to be affected by spinal disc problems more than men, which may seem surprising, as traditionally men have been the ones to carry heavier physical loads. We shouldn't assume that greater physical effort will automatically lead to a herniated disc.

Here's an interesting observation: cases of low back pain in patients who are receiving occupational health and safety benefits following an accident in the workplace often take longer to treat—because of the psychological factor, I suspect. When a patient feels like a victim, it's only natural for them to want their wrongs to be righted fairly. Unfortunately this doesn't always happen, and that's when anger, bitterness, and frustration can come into the picture and complicate things. In my practice, I see a lot of trivial sprains that have persisted because of the stress suffered by patients who have experienced an accident—in the workplace or elsewhere.

WHEN AUTHORITY BECOMES A PAIN IN THE NECK

Emotions also wield a heavy sword over the vulnerable area of the neck. I've observed that patients who have problems with authority have a propensity to present with neck pain and headaches. There are plenty of books out there that suggest psychosomatic connections like these are the body's way of telling us something.[18] As with everything in life, we should take this food for thought about our ailments and emotions with a pinch of salt and filter out what doesn't fit with our experience. But I have treated neck pain in employees who felt overpowered by their boss, as well as in teenagers with overbearing parents, or even patients who have had run-ins with the government—being lumbered with an income tax notice, for instance—or the police. Basically, I've often observed a connection between neck problems and a difficulty dealing with authority. After all, the neck is what supports the head, and the head is the part of the body that represents authority.

The neck is probably one of the parts of the body most vulnerable to psychological tension. Most of us suffer from some fatigue in the muscles that support the neck and head, as well as the shoulder muscles, because of the constant effects of stress. When people are under stress, it's common to see them with hunched shoulders—sometimes so high up toward their ears that pushing down on their shoulders will lower them by a good inch or two! Whenever our shoulders are lifted by psychological stress, the muscle is contracted, and it ultimately will become painful. It's important to move our neck and shoulders and be aware of stress so we can ward off painful neck tension.

WHEN TENSION GOES TO YOUR HEAD

It can't be overstated just how significant a role stress and overwork play in the occurrence of migraines. I've lost count of how many times I've heard people say they couldn't wait to get home on Friday night and relax after a rough week at work or in their personal life, only a few hours later to feel the first signs of a migraine coming on that ended up ruining their entire weekend! Incidentally, menstruation increases women's chances of getting a migraine, because it's a time of instability due to fluctuating hormones.

STRESS AND HEART PAIN

We know today that the heart is a particularly sensitive organ that reacts to essentially everything that's going on in our body. The slightest heartbeat can reflect what we're feeling inside, and there's not a single movement that isn't imbued with our emotions. Researchers have discovered that there are more nerve fibers in the heart than muscle fibers, as well as more magnetic electricity radiating from the heart than from the brain. That's the kind of discovery no one can ignore. Finally we're being told some good news about our hearts.

Now we need to shift our focus to the *role* our heart plays, or should play. I have previously written about broken-heart syndrome—the affectionate term for **takotsubo cardiomyopathy**, a condition that can cause symptoms of chest pain like a mild heart attack. The incidence of this condition is particularly high in women who are under significant stress. Conversely, men's hearts are particularly sensitive to anger, which is said to increase the risk of heart disease or death by up to 200 percent.[19]

INFLAMMATION, STRETCHED LIGAMENTS, stationary positions, long hours in front of a computer screen, and intense exercise without adequate preparation can all be triggers for musculoskeletal pain. We've also seen how negative emotions and stress can generate these same types of pain. However, there are certain types of pain and illness that stem primarily from poor lifestyle choices. As far as lifestyle goes, food is a key factor in understanding the causes of inflammation, and proper nutrition can be a major ally when it comes to preventing and treating chronic pain and illness. This is what we'll be exploring in the next chapter.

CHAPTER 4

Pain Treatment Starts on Your Plate

||||||||||||||||||||||||||||||||||||||||||||||||||||||||||||||||||

Let food be thy medicine and medicine be thy food.

HIPPOCRATES

I**T'S BECOMING MORE** and more clear just how essential a role proper nutrition and adequate gut flora have to play in keeping us healthy. This chapter on nutrition is fundamental reading, because it outlines some of the latest revelations about the connections between our food and our health. The more research and studies progress, the more we realize—to our great surprise—that we can relieve and even heal chronic ailments with the food we eat. Food can be both treatment and prevention, since the two go hand in hand. And it has a domino effect on our health: in trying to resolve a localized problem, we'll benefit our entire body.

There's no doubt that what we ingest constantly shapes both our physical and mental health. It would be naive to think that what we put into our cells every day has no effect on our well-being, or lack thereof. Just like the planet has started to react in a troubling way to the garbage and pollution we humans have been dumping on it for years, the food we've modified and tampered with in the name of improving its shelf life, appearance, and taste is perilously eating away at the health of the human body. There's only so much the body can take, and it's not surprising that sickness is ever more present in our lives in spite of our supposed advances in pharmaceuticals and technology.

So, why have there been all these changes—in our environment as well as in our personal eating habits?

Addicted to sugar

Starting around the mid-1960s,[1] people were urged to embrace the new "fat-free" diet touted by so-called expert authorities. Their intention was to nip cardiovascular disease in the bud, yet here we are now stuck in the worst epidemic of obesity and heart disease the world has ever known.[2] How did it all go wrong? Well, as we reduced our fat intake, we increased our sugar intake.[3] Of course, we had to eat *something*, right?

Nowadays, sugar is everywhere. Nearly three out of four products in our grocery store aisles contain significant quantities of sugar, so it's not surprising that over the last fifty years, we've unconsciously tripled our consumption. According to Statistics Canada, Canadians' total annual sugar intake has increased from 25 to nearly 70 kilograms (55 to almost 155 pounds), an increase mostly attributable to the various types of sugars added to processed foods. It's the same story in the United States as well—according to the federal government's *Dietary Guidelines* for 2015-2020, the average American consumes seventeen teaspoons of added sugars per day![4]

Many manufacturers add sugar to their products to heighten the flavor—but it's not only added sugar that's a problem. Until recently, nutrition recommendations like Canada's Food Guide and the USDA Food Guide Pyramid advised that the foundation of our diet should be made up of carbs like bread, pasta, and grains—a source of sugar in disguise, because they turn into sugars when we digest them. Over-consumption of fruit also adds to our sugar load, especially when it's in liquid form: sweet fruit juice is easy to knock back, but drinking too much of it sends our system out of whack. Even though the sugar in fruit is natural, it's still sugar, so we mustn't eat it to excess. (The health recommendation to aim for five to eight portions of fruit and vegetables per day should really be four to six portions of vegetables per day and one to two portions of fruit.)

The effects of all this sugar can manifest in a variety of ways. If you suffer from bulimia, hunger pangs, fatigue, or irritability, sugar may well be to blame. Sugar is also one of the most addictive products on the market; even lab rats get addicted to sugar and prefer it to cocaine.[5] Many of us love the taste of it so much that we refuse to give it up even as it silently wreaks havoc on our system.

It's not surprising, then, that as a society, we're growing more obese, diabetic, cardiac, arthritic, cancerous, and inflammatory than ever. It's not fat per se that's causing us to gain weight, but rather too much sugar. Unless we're constantly burning energy through exercise or sustained physical effort, which isn't the case for most of us, the body will convert sugar into fat reserves, which spread throughout our tissue, our blood, and even our organs—particularly the liver.

RESISTANT TO INSULIN

Many of us have levels of insulin (the hormone that reduces blood sugar) that are elevated two to three times above normal, if not higher. We know today that these elevated insulin levels are conducive to greater inflammation and a higher incidence of obesity.[6] And wherever there's inflammation, pain and disease are never far away. When sugar increases our insulin levels—even if our blood sugar is within a normal range—it can still cause a lot of damage and create a domino effect of inflammation. In most cases, reducing our sugar intake will reduce the spikes and fluctuations in our insulin levels and bring them back to normal.

Even having a slightly high level of blood sugar, as we find in people with mild diabetes, can be conducive to many chronic illnesses—such as dementia, cancer, depression, and heart disease—and the chronic pain associated with various inflammatory conditions. China, Africa, and India are expected to see a 60 to 120 percent increase in the incidence of diabetes in the next few years. Diabetes is a social disease and a very real pandemic.

SUGAR AND YOUR LIVER

Speaking of the liver, **hepatic steatosis** is one silent disease we rarely hear about. Commonly known as fatty liver, this disease fills the liver with fat cells that compress the healthy cells. This makes the liver swell, preventing it from doing its job to detoxify the body. The hepatic enzymes become too elevated, effectively overloading the liver and potentially causing discomfort in the abdomen, fatigue, and swelling in the legs. If the condition persists, the liver may become depleted, which may ultimately lead to cirrhosis—a disease that can be fatal. Cirrhosis has traditionally been thought of as a disease affecting people with alcohol addiction (when you think about it, alcohol does contain a lot of calories and sugar!). But today, more and more cases of hepatic steatosis are being observed even in in patients who drink very little alcohol. Excess sugar and diabetes are both contributing factors to this increase, as well as to a rise in cases of heart disease.

Eat well for your health

Dr. Mark Hyman, director of the Cleveland Clinic's Center for Functional Medicine and chairman of the board of the Institute for

Functional Medicine (IFM), is a strong advocate for healthy eating and its beneficial effects on chronic illnesses. In his book *Eat Fat, Get Thin*, he talks about not only the preventive aspects of a healthy, balanced diet, but also its curative powers.[7] It's not about counting calories, he maintains—no more excusing sugar because it's lower in calories than fat—but about nutritional quality above all else. Thanks to new findings in biochemical science and medicine, we now know we were wrong to cut fats in general—except for harmful trans fats— out of our diet. Science has shown us that there is far more to nutrition than simply consuming calories; food feeds information into our cells and DNA, too.

That's right: what we eat can even change our genetic makeup, as the exciting new field of nutrigenomics is revealing. Studies on the agouti mouse illustrate this principle well: under the influence of a specifically designed diet, this yellow-coated rodent, which carries an obesity gene, slimmed down remarkably and developed a brown coat instead. Another example from nature is the humble worker bee. When fed exclusively royal jelly, it becomes a queen, doubling in size and boosting its life expectancy from five months to five years! Who ever said nutrition had nothing to do with genetics?

It's time to throw that plate of too much sugar and too little fat right in the garbage. The traditional food pyramid dating from 1992 and 2007, with grains, bread, and pasta at its base, is now crumbling under the weight of the harmful diseases plaguing our society. A brand-new version of Canada's Food Guide was published in 2018, heralding some long-awaited changes. As well as encouraging us all to drink more water, the new guidelines recommend we eat a wide range of vegetables and fruit, protein-rich foods, and whole grains. Gone is the idea of food groups, and there are no more specific ref- erences to milk, dairy products, and meat and meat alternatives. There is no more talk about portions and quantities; instead, the focus is on filling our plates with variety, color, and freshness. It cer- tainly is refreshing to see recommendations that encourage us to eat healthily and remind us how easy this can be. That's not all: the new recommendations encourage us to take the time to enjoy our food, cook more, dine in good company, and be mindful of how much we eat, as well as reducing our intake of salt, sugar, and saturated fats. It's nice to see the government making healthy habits a part of the conversation about healthy eating.

And so, the ancient food pyramid is becoming a thing of the past. It's starting to make way for a new, healthier plate filled with plenty of vegetables of all kinds and colors; whole foods (including whole grains); and plenty of good fats, including eggs, fish rich in omega-3s, coconut oil, walnuts, avocados (as often as possible), extra-virgin olive oil, and even organic butter. And while some sugar can certainly be part of our diet, we should be minimizing it to make more room for protein and good fats. This nutritional realignment is a welcome corrective to the outdated diet of the past decades; it will reset the balance and change our health for the better.

HEALTHY FATS FOR THE BRAIN

Good fats are essential for our physical and psychological well-being. A deficiency in healthy fat can lead to imbalances at many levels: hormonal, immune, digestive, cutaneous, cerebral, or emotional. Because the brain is made up primarily of fat and water, diets low in fat and high in sugar have increased the frequency of dementia, especially Alzheimer's disease. We should listen to our inner caveman and embrace more of a hunter-gatherer approach to our food—with plenty of protein and fat, lots of vegetables, and some fruit—and a greater balance of activity in our lifestyle.

I'M GOING TO turn the next few pages of this book over to nutritionist Natasha Azrak, who trained at McGill University and co-founded the Clinique VI health practice outside Montreal. She is Canada's first nutritionist to be certified by the Institute for Functional Medicine, and Dr. Hyman himself calls her a "Health Warrior." Read on to learn more about the nutritional habits we should be adopting to

minimize the inflammatory process and reduce joint pain and inflammation in tendons and ligaments. Recognized by leading authorities
in functional medicine, Azrak's approach is proving to have undeni-
able benefits when it comes to chronic illness and pain. What's more,
the topics of nutrition and imbalance of the intestinal flora are on
everyone's lips right now in the enlightened medical community. It's
a fascinating subject, as you will see.

The diet–pain connection

By Natasha Azrak, Nutritionist, RD, IFMCP

PAIN IS CONNECTED to inflammation, and that's why the medical treatments recommended for pain often involve taking anti-inflammatories. But what's the connection between inflammation and nutrition? To what extent can the food we eat play a role in the inflammatory process that's generating so much pain and sickness these days? After all, many foods and nutrients, such as capsaicin (the active component of chili peppers), sulforaphane (found in broccoli), polyphenols, and phytonutrients are known for having the same biochemical effects as anti-inflammatory drugs.

These were the things I wanted to learn about when I decided to study nutrition at university. I wanted to find nutritional solutions for the migraines, digestive pain, and fatigue I'd been suffering from since childhood. I had experienced a lot of frustration due to these ailments because I didn't feel understood. I had consulted one doctor after another, and all the tests I underwent came back "normal." I was prescribed medications and various exercises, but nothing really worked, and often something that was supposed to solve the problem ended up making it worse. My grandmother would always make mint tea to help ease my digestive pains, so I have her to thank for piquing my curiosity and inspiring me to learn about the connections between nutrition, pain, and overall health.

It was in the Clinical Nutrition Level 2 course in my fourth year of studies that the topic of digestive illnesses and remedies finally came up. Much to my disappointment, the conclusion was that there was still no proof of any connection between nutrition and those illnesses. I had been so excited thinking I would finally get to the bottom of my problem, and I had worked so hard to get to that point—I couldn't believe there was no connection there. I figured I would go on to do a doctorate in naturopathy in Toronto.

But then I met Dr. Brouillard, and he suggested I explore the path of functional medicine instead. He explained that the problem with the various health professions—medicine, nutrition, and naturopathy alike—was that teaching methods were focused on the ailment itself rather than on health and prevention. In medicine, the goal is to find the right diagnosis as quickly and effectively as possible in order to prescribe treatment for the ailment that is diagnosed. In naturopathy, natural products are often used to manage the symptoms of an ailment, but the approach is still very much focused on the manifestations of a problem and not its causes. And in the field of nutrition, too, what I learned during my undergraduate degree revolved around different types of diet for different ailments (a diet for reflux, a diet for high blood pressure, a diet for cholesterol—you get the picture). In the case of reflux, for example, changing the patient's diet by cutting out tomatoes, coffee, juice, and alcohol will quickly make the symptoms go away. However, if the patient reintroduces one of those foods and the reflux then returns, it means the cause of the problem hasn't been eliminated, and the patient will have to remain on the special diet over the long term to relieve their symptoms.

Functional medicine, by contrast, aims to understand the source of a patient's symptoms. Often, the cause of reflux is either the presence of a type of bacteria called *Helicobacter pylori (H. pylori)* in the stomach or else a lack of gastric acidity.[8] Rather than trying to find a diet that works or a natural or pharmaceutical antacid to relieve the problem, in functional medicine we try to pinpoint what's causing the problem. Once we eliminate the bacteria or restore the proper acidity, the patient won't need to take supplements, follow a special diet, or take medication over the long term, because the problem will be solved. Functional medicine is all about this personalized, investigative approach to finding out *why* the symptoms are present. For instance, the causes of a patient's pain may be related to a digestive or hormonal imbalance, and functional medicine will strive to correct that imbalance primarily through food. If need be, it will resort to natural supplements to accelerate the corrective process and restore the patient's autonomy in terms of health—to ensure the patient won't have to rely forever on a diet, supplements, or drugs to manage their symptoms.

It didn't take long for me to decide to train for my certification in functional medicine. And nothing was going to stop me—not time, nor money. I was desperate to finally understand why I was having these problems. As I write these words today, I'm proud to be the first and only nutritionist certified in functional medicine in Canada. But I'm even more proud to say that that I've found the answers to my questions; I no longer suffer from migraines or digestive pain, and I even have more energy than I did as a child. It's incredible what a difference this has made to my life, and I'd like to share some of the wisdom I've gained.

Let's start with the basics when it comes to the connection between nutrition and inflammation. As we saw earlier, some foods have anti-inflammatory properties. Simply consuming these will make a difference in the short term, but a functional medicine approach will help us to find out what's causing the inflammation in the first place.

THE BACTERIA OUR HEALTH DEPENDS ON

The digestive system is our largest organ, and it makes up 60 percent of the body. If we include all the bacteria it contains, it represents some 90 percent of our cells!

In turn, 90 percent of these cells are bacteria. In the great scheme of things, our bodies are essentially carriers for these tiny organisms. We might think that our immune system's role is to protect us from bacteria, but in fact it depends on them to keep us safe. Amazingly, our digestive system encounters the same number of foreign bodies in a single day as our immune system encounters in an entire lifetime![9] This means that our digestive system is our first line of defense against invaders. Digestive flora play a key role in providing this protection, because good bacteria are always the first to attack bad bacteria. Unfortunately, not all of us have a healthy intestinal flora.

If our intestinal flora is inadequate, the shortage of good bacteria makes us more vulnerable to bad bacteria. Several studies have shown that North Americans and Europeans harbor more harmful bacteria than Africans, because of their food, lifestyle, and birthing methods, among other reasons.

When we have more bad bacteria in our body than good, we call this **dysbiosis**. Dysbiosis disrupts the partnership between our microbiota and immune system, leading to altered immune responses that may underlie various inflammatory disorders. Studies have shown how dysbiosis can be at the root of a wide range of illnesses: inflammatory intestinal diseases such as ulcerative colitis, Crohn's disease, and diverticulitis; immune diseases, including asthma and skin disorders (psoriasis, eczema, hives, acne); autoimmune diseases such as multiple sclerosis, and even metabolic disorders such as diabetes and obesity. If you never seem to be able to lose your abdominal fat, inadequate flora may in fact be the reason. A number of studies suggest this, including one carried out in Canada.[10] Farmers have known for years that administering antibiotics to animals (which destabilizes their flora), even in small doses, stimulates their growth and fattens them up, much to their economic benefit. Why would it be any different for humans? And abdominal fat produces a number of inflammatory hormones, which can aggravate the condition of a patient struggling with pain.

That's why, if you're experiencing digestive symptoms—even if they're not very problematic (such as occasional constipation, diarrhea, bloating, or gas), and even if you've had tests done and your physician tells you the results show nothing is wrong, or gives you the default diagnosis of irritable bowel syndrome—it's important to pay attention to the state of your digestive system. As you can see, it's the guardian of your health in so many ways!

A number of factors are favorable to a healthy flora:

1) Being born by vaginal delivery (not by C-section).
This ensures a base level of flora that will always be there as a foundation, regardless of what we eat.[11]

2) Being breastfed.
It takes at least six months to a year of breastfeeding to build healthy flora in a baby.[12]

3) A healthy diet.
What you eat has only a short-term impact on your flora, affecting it for about a week—hence the importance of making a healthy diet an ongoing part of your lifestyle. Consuming foods known as **probiotics** and **prebiotics** stimulates the reproduction of good bacteria.

The variety and quality of your diet is equally important. The more varied your diet, the more diverse your flora will be. Here's a simple tip: try to get all the colors of the rainbow on your plate every day. Challenge yourself to step out of your dietary comfort zone! Turning this exercise into a game at the grocery store is a great way to teach kids healthy eating habits, too: ask them to find a vegetable of every color to put in your shopping basket. The more children are in contact with vegetables and help with choosing them, the more familiar those vegetables will be on their plate.

As for food quality, there's evidence that many artificial sweeteners, such as aspartame, sucralose, and saccharin, alter the digestive flora.[13] This is why switching from drinking regular cola to diet cola can make your diabetes worse,[14] because gut flora is such an important part of our health. The best sugar substitute is a plant called stevia. Just like mint, it grows like a weed, and like mint, when it's dried it has a pleasant taste and will keep all year. Xylitol can also be used, but only in small quantities, as ingesting large quantities can cause diarrhea.

PROBIOTICS AND PREBIOTICS

There's more to **probiotics** than the supplements you see in the health-food store! Fermented foods contain probiotics too. Fermenting food is a culinary tradition that transcends cultures around the world, but in North America it has largely become a lost art. In Europe and the Middle East, probiotics are widespread in foods such as yogurt, sauerkraut, and pickled vegetables such as olives. Many commercial yogurts no longer contain sufficient quantities of bacteria, however; the bacteria they do contain have some impact, but not as much as the bacteria in home-made yogurt, which is still live. Homemade yogurt is surprisingly easy to make—there are plenty of recipes on the internet if you feel like trying it for yourself. Aged cheeses, sourdough bread, kefir, and kombucha (fermented tea) are also good sources of active bacteria, as are foods of Asian origin such as kimchi (fermented cabbage) and natto, miso, and tempeh, all made from fermented soybeans.

Prebiotics are types of dietary fiber that feed the bacteria in the gut. Whereas probiotics stimulate the reproductive process of the flora—I like to think of them as cheerleaders—prebiotics are the food needed for the flora to reproduce. This is why taking probiotics along with a low-fiber diet won't have the beneficial effect you are looking for. Sources of prebiotic fiber include onion, garlic, shallots, asparagus, chicory, Jerusalem artichoke, pumpkin, and almonds.

4) Avoiding antibiotics as much as possible.

After you take antibiotics, it can take two years to restore your flora through your diet if you don't take steps to help matters along. You can imagine the consequences on a generation of children who were prescribed antibiotics every time they complained of an earache or tonsillitis! This practice has greatly altered their immune defenses, and some experts are now wondering whether it may be the cause of the epidemic of ailments we're seeing today, such as intestinal disorders, food allergies and intolerances, weakened immune resistance, and an increased incidence of autoimmune diseases.

Even if you haven't taken antibiotics for several years, you may have come into contact with them all the same if the animals whose meat you eat were given antibiotics. That's why it's important to choose organic meat and dairy, which have the added bonus of being better for the environment.[15]

We've touched on the various factors that can have a negative impact on digestive flora. Another reason it's important to maintain a balanced intestinal flora is that dysbiosis—having more bad bacteria than good—can lead to a leaky gut.

WHAT IS A LEAKY GUT?

The intestine has a lining made up of layer upon layer of cells that only let fully digested food into the bloodstream. When we have dysbiosis, the good bacteria don't protect our intestinal lining, so holes can develop between these cells, allowing food that hasn't been fully digested to leak out. This is referred to as **leaky gut syndrome**. The problem is that when these larger food molecules pass through the digestive cells into the bloodstream to nourish the other cells in the body, the immune system, which is constantly on the lookout for foreign bodies, doesn't recognize the undigested material and has to decide whether or not to attack the intruder. If it attacks, this is called a **food intolerance**.

Let's take a moment to clarify what a food intolerance actually is, since the term is tending to be used with an increasingly broad interpretation. There are three types of situation that warrant the term "intolerance":

1) Enzyme deficiency

Lactose intolerance is one example that falls into this category. This kind of intolerance is due to the digestive system, not the immune system—it's not created by food passing through holes in the intestinal lining, as described above. Instead, the problem stems from a lack of lactase enzymes, which break down lactose sugars. This deficiency is often genetic, and adding the enzyme when consuming lactose can resolve the problem.

2) Allergies

Gluten allergy, known as celiac disease, has been frequently misunderstood and is often confused with gluten intolerance. It's now become clear, though, that it's possible to be gluten intolerant without necessarily being allergic. There is a difference, and it's very important to understand.

As with peanut allergy, the cause of gluten allergy is unknown. But once the body has "memorized" the allergy, it's there for life, and a tiny molecule is all it takes to trigger a reaction. This means that if you're allergic to gluten, putting gluten-free bread in a toaster that has been in contact with bread made from wheat will be just as harmful as eating bread that contains gluten! The symptoms of gluten allergy and peanut allergy are very different, however. Peanuts often set off an anaphylactic response, which is a very serious reaction manifesting as hives, swelling in the throat and lungs, a drop in blood pressure, heart arrhythmia, breathing difficulty, and possibly cardiac arrest. By contrast, gluten allergy triggers an attack on the digestive cells. It's considered an autoimmune disease because when an allergic person's immune system comes into contact with a gluten molecule, it attacks their own cells.

Gluten allergy can be difficult to detect because not everyone experiences the same symptoms. Most people assume that celiac disease presents as a host of digestive issues. However, some people may experience it instead as a form of anemia that won't respond to taking iron supplements (because the digestive cells are under attack, iron is not absorbed properly). Others may show no symptoms at all.

It's recently become very much in vogue to follow a gluten-free diet, but before eliminating gluten from your diet, it's important to check whether you're actually allergic. This is why some doctors suggest that all new patients should be tested for potential gluten allergy. If you've already eliminated gluten from your diet of your own accord, without being tested first, you're likely to see a false negative on the test. You'll have to reintroduce gluten to your diet (typically two slices of bread or one cup of pasta per day) for at least three weeks before doing the test to ensure an accurate result. If you haven't done the test but really don't want to reintroduce gluten into your diet because the symptoms are too severe, the HLA DQ2 and DQ8 genetic test may be an option. This doesn't require you to consume gluten, and if the result is negative, you'll never develop the allergy. However, if the test is positive, that does not necessarily mean that you're allergic, but that you could be (the test identifies a gene, and only about 15 percent of people with this gene develop celiac disease). In this case, you must then do the blood test—and eat gluten for three weeks beforehand—to either confirm or rule out the allergy. If the result is negative, from that point on you won't have to worry as much about minor gluten contamination.

3) Intolerances

Intolerances are very different from allergies. They're also not a figment of the imagination! If people feel better when they cut out gluten, it isn't just in their minds. They might not be allergic as such, but the intolerance is real.[16] In fact, the symptoms are caused by a leaky gut (the holes between the cells we talked about earlier).[17] When digested food passes through these holes, the immune system memorizes that food; then every time it encounters that food, the immune system creates antibodies[18] and inflammation, which results in pain.

As a result, the foods to which we're most intolerant may often be the foods we eat most frequently. That would explain why we point the finger at gluten and dairy products so often, because they're some of the most common foods in the North American diet. The thing is, it's not necessarily these foods that are to blame, but rather the holes in the intestine that are making the food we eat problematic. Many patients come to see me and tell me how they cut out gluten or dairy and felt better in the beginning, but the pain gradually returned and now they feel they're reacting to more and more foods. The reason for this is that they simply eliminated certain foods without addressing the cause of the problem (the holes in the intestine). If you have a leaky gut, it's the foods you eat the most often that will come into contact with your immune system. There's not necessarily a connection with the quality of the food itself. Even the healthiest foods, like spinach and broccoli, may be problematic for you if that's what you put on your plate most often.

The good news is that unlike with allergies, if you have an intolerance your immune system produces antibodies that only have a short memory (three to six months). When you eliminate these foods and plug the leaks, these foods can often be reintroduced later without causing any problems. That's the whole idea of an elimination diet.[19] When you follow this type of diet, you eliminate the foods you eat the most often (for instance, gluten, corn, dairy products, soy, eggs, and beef). The diet typically lasts for thirty days. Then you reintroduce the foods you eliminated one by one to see which ones are problematic for you. If any foods cause problems, you'll then have to wait three to six months before introducing them again to see whether they're still intolerable. I should stress that the idea of this diet isn't to lose weight—it's important not to eat less or limit your portions. And remember, if the leaks aren't plugged, other intolerances may emerge. Another thing to bear in mind is that these elimination diets can be very difficult to follow and can create significant vitamin and mineral imbalances. This is why it's important to follow a diet like this under proper guidance and for as short a time as possible (only until the leaks are plugged).

The other good news is that, as opposed to allergies, intolerances aren't triggered by trace amounts. Because the reaction you experience is proportionate to the quantity of the food you consumed, it can sometimes be very difficult to pinpoint what's causing the intolerance—hence the importance of reintroducing only one food at a time when the time comes. You also won't need to replace your toaster if you discover that you're simply gluten intolerant rather than allergic, because any reaction to remnants of gluten stuck in the toaster will be minimal. Similarly, minimal quantities of gluten in sauces and marinades are unlikely to cause many symptoms, whereas if you're truly allergic, these traces of gluten will cause your immune system to attack your digestive cells even if you don't feel any great symptoms.

When there are leaks to plug in your gut, the greatest challenge for your body is that it has to treat so many once-familiar foods and sources of energy as enemies. Your body gets confused and starts sending out distress signals by creating inflammation. Our immune system is active throughout our body, which keeps us safe but also explains how inflammatory disorders can be so widespread in our organ systems—from rheumatoid arthritis, osteoarthritis, and spondylitis in our bones to ulcerative colitis, Crohn's disease, and diverticulitis in our digestive system to psoriasis on our skin.

These are some of the conditions associated with a leaky gut:
- Food intolerances
- Migraines
- Gallstones (cholelithiasis)
- Chronic fatigue syndrome
- Various autoimmune diseases: type 1 diabetes, celiac disease, rheumatoid arthritis, psoriasis, Hashimoto's thyroiditis

The effects may even extend to cardiovascular disease, as several studies[20] are now suggesting that that the inflammation from a leaky gut may be a potential factor in the development of atherosclerosis (a disease in which fat deposits build up inside the arteries).

How do you know if you have a leaky gut? There may be various symptoms, including slow digestion, difficulty digesting protein or fat, the presence of food or oil particles in your stools, malodorous stools or flatulence, constipation, and diarrhea. However, many people may exhibit none of these symptoms and still have a leaky gut.

What causes these leaks? As we've already seen, inadequate gut flora is one of the factors. Alcohol consumption is another, as is endurance running. Stress is a significant factor, too, so worrying about what you will or won't be able to eat can make the problem worse if you don't have the proper support while you're following a restrictive diet.

THE 5RS APPROACH

What's the best way to digest all of this information? As we've just learned, many factors can come into play with inflammatory disorders. And as stated earlier, the goal of functional medicine is to solve the problem at its source and not treat only the symptoms. In functional medicine, we use a step system called the **5Rs** to eliminate inflammation. A professional trained in this approach can help you go through the process.

1. Remove:
a. Bad bacteria, parasites, yeast (this will require investigation and medical treatment)
b. Foods that cause intolerance

Removing the stressors means getting rid of things that negatively affect the environment of the gastrointestinal tract, including foods, parasites, and other harmful microorganisms, such as bacteria and yeast. This might involve using an elimination diet.

2. Replace (any deficiencies):
a   Vitamin D
b. Fiber
c. Omega-3s
d. Zinc
e. Magnesium
f. Potassium

This step involves correcting nutritional deficiencies that may hinder proper bodily function by adding nutrients to the diet such as vitamin D and zinc, which are required by the immune system; fiber, which is important for the digestive system; and omega-3s, which are natural anti-inflammatories.

3. Reinoculate (with):
a. Probiotics
b. Prebiotics

The goal here is to reinoculate the digestive flora—as explained earlier, with probiotics (live bacteria that stimulate the reproduction of flora) and prebiotics (fiber that feeds the bacteria so they can reproduce).

4. Repair (with):
a. Glutamine

To plug the leaks in the gut, we have to provide the necessary nutrients, such as the amino acid glutamine, for the cells to reproduce quickly. A word of caution: some people may have a reaction to glutamine, which is often a sign that a step has been missed and that bad bacteria are still present.

5. Rebalance:
a. Diet
b. Physical activity
c. Sleep
d. Stress
e. Avoid unnecessary antibiotics

If we want to reap long-term benefits and prevent recurrence, it's essential to adopt healthy life habits to correct the lifestyle imbalance that caused the problem in the first place. Avoid antibiotics at all costs if you don't need them. For instance, if you have a viral rather than a bacterial infection, there's no point taking antibiotics—rest will do the trick! If you do need to take antibiotics, be sure to take the probiotic *Saccharomyces boulardii* throughout the course of your treatment. Because it's a type of fungus, not bacteria, it won't be affected by the antibiotics that are killing the bacteria in your body—good and bad—and it will provide protection during your treatment. Once the course of treatment is over, choose a variety of strains of probiotics containing the *Lacto* and *Bifido* families.

It's important not to do these steps out of order—for instance, the treatment may not work if you do the second R, reinoculating the bacteria, when you still have a lot of bad bacteria, as you might feed them and encourage them to multiply and grow.

I first encountered Karina five years ago. At that time, she was very sick. She was suffering from vasculitis, a disease characterized by the immune system attacking the blood vessels. In her case, the blood vessels in her legs were affected to the point that her skin in that area would often bleed and get infected, secreting pus. She didn't understand what was happening and tried to find a doctor. The first doctor she saw told her it was an allergy, and another told her it was nothing serious and she shouldn't worry.

Finally, she found a doctor who told her she had the worst case of vasculitis he had ever seen! Following her diagnosis, Karina underwent chemotherapy treatments and took steroids and medication. These depleted her immune system and caused many side effects, including a risk of developing cancer because her immune system had been suppressed. She tried everything and even explored some experimental treatments.

Karina was able to walk and she was in less pain, but her body was no longer functioning normally. She was no longer able to think clearly, her muscles hurt incredibly, and she was so tired that she could barely do anything in a day—despite the fact, she told me, that she used to be so full of energy before her illness. Just as she was beginning to lose hope, a friend of hers told her about our clinic.

When Karina came to the practice, she told me she couldn't go on living the way she was. It just didn't make sense to her. At twenty-seven years old, she was taking twenty-three different drugs, with countless side effects. Karina chose to place her trust in me and in functional medicine. She thought the idea sounded different and interesting and it made so much sense to her, as she had taken many antibiotics in her childhood and had had many years of stress and irregular eating habits before she got sick.

And so we applied the 5Rs approach. The first R—Remove—was intended to determine whether she had dysbiosis (a poor balance of flora). Various types of stool analysis can provide this information. This first step also involved removing all foods that might be causing an intolerance, so I prescribed an elimination diet for Karina (see above for details).

The second R—Replace—consisted of replacing what was missing. We first made sure Karina had enough vitamin D in her bloodstream. We enriched her diet with omega-3s and minerals, and we focused on giving her some good sources of fiber to start nourishing her flora. This was depleted because Karina had taken vast quantities of antibiotics during her childhood, and she was experiencing a number of digestive symptoms.

Then came the third R—Reinoculate. We used probiotic supplements and introduced fermented foods. The fiber we had already integrated into Karina's diet served as prebiotics.

For step 4—Repair—we prescribed a daily dose of 15 grams of glutamine, because leaky gut syndrome is so prevalent in cases of autoimmune diseases.

The fifth and final R—Rebalance—involved maintaining a varied diet, after reintroducing foods one by one to check which ones were problematic for Karina. We also paid attention to the other systems of her body.

Going through this process improved Karina's skin and her energy to the point that the physician who was treating her autoimmune disease began trials to dial back her medication. This happened very gradually based on the improvement in the appearance of Karina's skin and her other symptoms.

Two years later, together with her physician, we managed to eliminate all twenty-three of the medications Karina had been taking. It's now been three years since she stopped taking immuno-suppressants completely, and her vasculitis has never returned. Karina's case is certainly a success story, as patients who are diagnosed with an autoimmune disease often have to take immunosuppressive drugs for life.

Today, Karina leads a normal life. She feels healthy and well nourished, and she loves the food she eats. She is now working and has her energy back. She can do everything she wants to do that she had to miss out on before. Everyone in her family has since decided to follow the same approach, too, even though their ailments were far from being as serious as hers. "There's always room to feel better!" they told me.

This story, and indeed all of the valuable information shared by Azrak above,[21] sums up the role of our digestive microbiota well. Clearly, it plays an essential part in maintaining our health and keeping chronic pain in check. In the pages ahead, we'll explore some other important topics related to diet and our health.

Take care of your teeth and gums

Just as new data is confirming the importance of the intestinal micro-biome, we are increasingly understanding the role of the microbiome upstream from the digestive system. If the microbiota (bacterial process) in the oral cavity is off balance, it may in turn make the other organs in the body sick. Gum disease such as gingivitis and the bone infection we call periodontitis promotes the incidence of heart disease, stroke, and even diabetes and arthritic diseases by generating and releasing these inflammatory cells into the bloodstream in great numbers.

That's why proper oral hygiene and dental visits to make sure our teeth and gums are healthy are an essential part of every proactive health routine. Brushing and flossing is a serious routine that should not be neglected. I often use a water-jet flosser as well, which does a good job of dislodging food particles. I also have my own recipe for keeping my gums healthy: I massage between my gums and teeth using a soft rubber toothpick that I dip in a 50/50 mixture of sea salt and baking soda (you can even add a dash of cinnamon if you like).

Go veggie or eat meat?

Ah, the age-old debate: what should we eat; what should we limit; and what should we cut out of our diet entirely? What is the ideal diet? Will vegetarianism end up ousting the traditional meat-based diet one day? I'm not a vegetarian, but I do believe that some people would benefit from eating a diet with less of a focus on meat. Generally speaking, vegetarianism is often associated with a more health-oriented lifestyle. That said, my medical experience has not suggested that vegetarians are always in better health than meat-eaters; I've detected dietary deficiencies in my vegetarian friends and in the most dedicated carnivores alike! But differences of opinion aside, there's another aspect to vegetarianism that should be considered.

We know that people belonging to traditional cultures that eat a mainly vegetarian diet consisting of whole foods and plants are much less prone to conditions associated with vascular damage. What's more, patients with recurrent cardiac disease that is so far advanced it's inoperable, advanced vascular lesions of the carotid arteries, arterial hypertension, and obesity have seen significant improvements to their health simply by embracing a vegetarian diet when medication and surgery could do nothing for them.

Arthur, a seventy-four-year-old male in Newfoundland, suffered a heart attack in 1982 at age forty-two, followed by a stroke three years later. His radiological scans confirmed that the right carotid artery was completely blocked and the left carotid artery had a 27 percent blockage. As well as being heavily medicated, Arthur made a modest change to his diet to eliminate sugar and fat and reduce his meat intake. In spite of changing his diet and adjusting his medication, Arthur's vascular problems continued to worsen, as is often the case. An ultrasound scan detected a new blockage, this time greater than 85 percent. In 2011, Arthur was experiencing angina attacks on a daily basis that forced him to become sedentary. His usual medication was no longer of any help to him.

Arthur's doctor and surgeon told him they had exhausted all the treatment options and could offer nothing more to him, as his condition was worsening further and further. Arthur was no longer able to look after himself at home, and he was living on borrowed time.

In the meantime, however, his daughter had heard about the Wellness Institute at the Cleveland Clinic in Ohio, because an associate at the clinic, Dr. Caldwell B. Esselstyn, Jr., had published a book entitled Prevent and Reverse Heart Disease.[22] *Arthur's daughter had suffered a heart attack herself at age thirty-seven, so she was serious about turning things around. She persuaded her father to try a new diet with her, this time under the guidance of Dr. Esselstyn. They both actively embraced this new natural, plant-based, whole-food diet, and after just one month, Arthur's angina issues had disappeared—as indeed had his erectile difficulties! Four months later, he had lost nearly 45 pounds and was back to the 130 or so pounds he weighed on his wedding day, fifty-three years earlier!*

By September 2013, his ultrasound scans confirmed the vascular occlusions in his carotid arteries had been reversed and were down from 85 to 60 percent! Today, Arthur is in great shape. He's full of energy and is busy living life to the fullest. And the thought of his days being numbered couldn't be further from his mind.

According to experts, a number of factors might explain these improvements. In some people, consuming meat, sugar, and milk can lead to a reduction in several beneficial blood enzymes. These foods can trigger a degradation of the intestinal microbiota and an increase in inflammation, which then spell the beginning of circulatory disorders and critical illnesses. Studies are continuing into diets that may not only prevent but also reverse vascular disease. Even though the results of these studies are not yet known, I need no convincing about the beneficial health effects and chronic pain relief of eating a good-quality diet and taking supplements. Obviously, Arthur's case is just one of many, and there are several factors that would need to be examined to prove the scientific merit of his diet. However, a number of similar cases have been reported, and it seems to show that this type of diet has many benefits to offer.

As the popularity of vegetarian diets continues to grow, recent scientific discoveries have highlighted its merits. Indeed, many of us could benefit from a diet richer in vegetables than the traditional meat-heavy fare to which North Americans have grown accustomed. Take the Mediterranean diet, for example. This mixed diet rich in vegetables, nuts, and fruit, but light on meat, has been shown to contribute to a significant reduction in incidences of heart disease.

Based on more than twenty-five years of studying patients in an advanced stage of cardiovascular disease, Dr. Esselstyn's research has found that a meat-free diet rich in vegetables and whole foods is conducive to vascular health. His research also suggests that it's not just about prevention, but also about improving and repairing the vascular tissue damaged by atherosclerosis (sclerosis of the arteries).

This is actually quite sensational, though it's not surprising that the medical community seems so skeptical about the healing power of a simple change in diet. I believe it's crucial for the medical community to recognize the therapeutic validity of nutrition. At a lecture I gave recently, two young medical students came forward to compliment me on my proactive approach that promotes nutrition and healthy life habits. I asked them what medical school had taught them about nutrition. They replied, with some dissatisfaction, that they had only had a few hours of teaching on the subject, and that the lecturer had ended the class with the words, "In any case, nutrition doesn't really matter, because we have drugs!"

On closer examination, we may wonder what Dr. Esselstyn's research means, besides demonstrating beyond the shadow of a doubt the harmful effects on some individuals of an excessively meat-heavy diet versus a vegetarian diet. How is it that vascular issues caused by atherosclerosis lesions that are aggravated by eating meat—with biochemical evidence to back it up—can be remedied by eating vegetarian? Hasn't the time come for us to understand all the implications of our dependency on food? Shouldn't we know by now that eating too much meat can ultimately undermine human health?

Most of us today will live past the age of eighty, and as we age, eating too much meat may result in an unhealthy buildup of fat deposits in our arteries, hindering the circulation that pumps blood all around our body—to our brain, our heart, and our limbs. We don't all have to become vegetarian, but we should reduce the quantity of meat we eat—a four- to six-ounce portion is sufficient, and we don't need to eat meat every day. Another benefit of eating less meat is that ultimately, it will reduce the number of animals that are raised for food and slaughtered, often in atrocious conditions.

THERE'S NO SUCH thing as a miracle diet. Instead, there are nutritional approaches that are appropriate for each circumstance and that can be tailored for each individual; there are excesses we can trim; and there is a more enlightened view of nutrition. It's clear that eating a healthy diet, with minimal amounts of inflammatory foods, plays an essential role when it comes to treating pain. We'll find out in the next chapter some other possible avenues for managing pain.

CHAPTER 5

Natural Pain-Relief Solutions

||||||||||||||||||||||||||||||||||||||||||||||||||||||||||||||||

The art of medicine consists of amusing
the patient, while nature cures the disease.

VOLTAIRE

W HAT CAN YOU do at home to relieve your pain and increase your sense of well-being? Here are some suggestions that might help improve your quality of life.

The power of natural supplements

||||||||||||||||||||||||||||||||||||||||||||||||||

Often it's possible to prevent inflammation or reduce pain with natural supplements. These offer the advantage of fewer side effects than prescription drugs; however, since they're not as concentrated, they can take longer to work and need to be taken for a longer period. If you're taking natural supplements and prescription drugs at the same time, it's a good idea to talk to a doctor who is aware of the issues. The interactions between different drugs can be difficult to evaluate, and the same goes for combining prescription drugs with supplements. If you mix a blue pill, a red pill, and a pink pill, how will that color your treatment?

Here's a list of natural products that may help reduce inflammation and keep pain under control. Their properties have not been tested by broad double-blind studies, but some research has shown they are effective and can offer benefits to many people struggling with pain and inflammation.

FIRST, TRIM THE EXCESS

Easing pain and reducing inflammation doesn't necessarily involve adding something new to your body. Sometimes it's better to remove something first! In fact, the first "natural supplement" you might want to try is simply abstinence. Before adding supplements, think about cutting down on things you don't need.

In our modern lifestyles, many of us have reduced our levels of physical activity without reducing our calorie intake accordingly. To maintain balance, those of us consuming more than we need may be able to cut back our food intake by up to 30 percent—while still making sure we're getting the right nutrients and not going hungry, of course. By simply trimming the excess, we can extend our life expectancy by several years, as some recent studies have shown.[1] The more we avoid overeating, the better it will be for our health, at least in our society of plenty where obesity is more of a problem than emaciation.

What should you cut out of your diet? The first step in recovering your health is to pass on unhealthy, high-calorie foods. Unfortunately, it's easier to pop a little pill than it is to cut out what's working against us. Kicking a habit we like is never fun, even if we know it's not good for us. Knowing something is not enough, and changes nothing in our lives; we have to take action. Only when we're truly convinced that a habit is bad for us and that it's making us suffer—and when we do something about it—can we finally make the change. Ultimately, pain is a mechanism that urges us to make a better choice. That said, we don't have to suffer, because we do have a choice. We can change our attitude and choose to make a change for our health instead of stagnating in illness and resistance.

LIVE FOR YOUR LIVER

Before beginning any treatment, you should also think about your faithful friend, your liver. Your liver is the biggest organ in your body and it has a remarkable capacity to regenerate itself. For example, with an organ donation, just a portion of the donor's liver can rebuild a whole liver in the recipient's body. Your liver is crucial to your gastrointestinal health, so why is it so often forgotten?

Your liver produces around two pints of bile every day to promote digestion. And that's not all—it manages and metabolizes 100,000 biochemical reactions every second and carries out 500 different essential functions for our survival and well-being. Everything you ingest must be metabolized by your liver. It's a champion at what it does, but we ask a lot of it, especially when we overdo things a little. It bends over backward for us, but it can start to drag its heels as we get older if we overload it with too much food, alcohol, drugs, and supplements day in, day out. Your liver sure could use a break sometimes!

More and more studies are reporting the benefits of partial intermittent fasting.[2] Occasionally abstaining from food for a sixteen-hour period—by skipping breakfast, for instance—can promote better hormone quality and enhance growth hormone secretion. This might be as simple as drinking lots of water with lemon instead of eating breakfast one day a week. It's not about following a restrictive diet— rather, it's about giving your digestive system a temporary reprieve. This kind of intermittent fasting can have positive impacts on your physiology and energy levels and become part of your lifestyle, not just a weight-loss strategy.

THE TOP GO-TO SUPPLEMENTS

Proteolytic enzyme supplements are natural substances that have proven their worth for decades for hundreds of millions of people struggling with pain in Europe, and more recently in Canada.[3] These digestive enzyme complexes are said to be a natural alternative to aspirin, helping with general circulatory issues and reducing pain and inflammation, particularly that due to osteoarthritis and other musculoskeletal ailments. Taken between mealtimes, these enzymes (brands include SpectraZyme, ProteoXyme, and Wobenzym) bolster the immune system and vascular system and reduce pain and inflammation by helping to digest harmful protein complexes in the bloodstream. They can be beneficial in reducing vascular issues like phlebitis—inflammation of a vein. A colleague told me how some hospitals in Germany use them on inpatients from the outset to avoid circulatory issues, including phlebitis and pulmonary embolisms. Note that pregnant women should abstain from these, as should individuals with coagulation disorders or liver complaints and anyone taking blood thinners.

Serrapeptase is another proteolytic enzyme (in other words, one that decomposes proteins). It controls inflammation by eliminating dead tissue, which can reduce arterial blockages. Serrapeptase promotes cardiovascular health and alleviates symptoms of arthritis by reducing inflammation and encouraging tissue repair.

Glucosamine and **chondroitin**, mainly used for inflammatory osteoarthritis, are known as **chondroprotectors**, because, as some studies suggest, they protect the cartilage. Their pain-relieving effect becomes apparent after one to two months of treatment. Because they have almost no side effects, these supplements can be taken over the long term. They seem to provide relief to more than 60 percent of people who use them. Why not try them and see if they work for you?

Resveratrol is a powerful antioxidant and anti-inflammatory.[4] We're hearing more and more about this beneficial substance found in red wine, berries, red grapes, peanuts, and certain plants. This isn't necessarily an endorsement of wine—many wines are treated with fungicides that destroy much of the resveratrol, which is why it's best to choose organic wines. But if you're looking for an effective dose of resveratrol, you should take it in supplement form. A glass of wine only contains 0.03 to 1.07 milligrams of resveratrol, which is not a therapeutic dose. By contrast, supplements provide a dosage of 50 to 100 mg per day, in the form of pills to be taken outside mealtimes. Resveratrol is an effective antioxidant that protects some elements (glutathione and mitochondria) responsible for giving us energy. It helps to preserve our DNA and contributes to greater longevity. When tested in animals, it's been shown to inhibit the formation of cancerous masses and even increase the effectiveness of chemotherapy drugs. It also promotes cardiovascular health by protecting the walls of the arteries. There's still a lot to discover about this fascinating molecule.

Collagen hydrolysate, or hydrolyzed collagen, is a substance derived from collagen that promotes the formation of new collagen, necessary for our connective and cartilage tissue. This supplement offers pain-relieving properties for the joints in general, assuming a sufficient dosage (typically 2,000 mg per day).

Valerian is used for its calming and stress-relieving properties. Together with **magnesium**, it can provide relief for individuals suffering from muscle tension, cramps, or spasms. What's more, magnesium is a mineral that has a calming effect on blood pressure.

Turmeric is a spice of Asian origin used widely in Indian and Chinese cuisine. It also deserves our full attention for its many beneficial properties, which include stimulating digestion by increasing bile secretion. Turmeric is your liver's friend, but be aware that if you have a biliary (bile duct) obstruction or kidney stones, you'd be wise to abstain or consult your physician before taking it. Turmeric also diminishes the bacteria *Helicobacter pylori*, which is responsible for stomach ulcers, and it's effective against a number of gastrointestinal disorders, including inflammatory intestinal diseases.

Some years ago, scientists isolated substances called **curcuminoids**—or curcumin—in the turmeric plant, which were found to have very powerful antioxidants and anti-inflammatory properties. Curcumin is known to relieve arthritis (at doses of up to 2 grams per day) and even provide general pain relief. Researchers are excited about its benefits on many levels. For example, curcumin inhibits cancerous cells and, in some cases, it has led to remarkable results in combination with chemotherapy. It's thought to have the power to reduce infection in general and to fight conditions including psoriasis, fibromyalgia, depression, and even some forms of dementia. Turmeric has a pleasant taste as well, so we have every reason to incorporate it into our daily diet. Curcumin is not very easily absorbed, however, and it's rapidly eliminated by the liver, so significant quantities are often necessary. As for its digestive properties, the World Health Organization has recognized its beneficial effects with doses as modest as 250 mg, four times a day. Curcumin absorption can be improved by taking it with black pepper and bromelain.

Omega-3s are a must in our daily diet. The benefits of these fatty acids—which include fish oils—have been widely documented for at least the last decade. As well as being used to improve cardiovascular health and memory, omega-3s are effective against diabetes, skin disorders, and depression, not to mention pain and inflammation. The primary components of omega-3s are DHA (docosahexaenoic acid) and EPA (eicosapentaenoic acid). EPA is the part that fights inflammation, assuming a dose of about 2 g per day. It works directly on the affected part of the body to reduce pain and inflammation in individuals suffering from rheumatoid arthritis. This shouldn't stop anyone else from eating good, fresh fish, though. I suggest whole sardines, a fish whose modest price is inversely proportional to its benefits!

THIAA (tetrahydro-iso-alpha acids) is a hops-derived extract that modulates pain by reducing inflammatory proteins (PGE2). A number of studies have shown this product to be effective at relieving joint pain. In some patients it acts like non-steroidal anti-inflammatory drugs (NSAIDs) without the unpleasant side effects that can include gastric issues.

Cilantro is an aromatic herb known to ease digestion and help eliminate heavy metals such as lead and mercury. Use it to add flair to any salad or a touch of greenery and burst of flavor to a range of dishes.

Finally, some other natural products with anti-inflammatory and pain-relieving properties to mention are **Boswellia serrata**, **ginger**, and **cat's claw**. Don't worry, this plant is gentler than it sounds!

Medical cannabis for pain relief

According to the UN, cannabis is the world's most commonly used drug, with some 200 million people said to use it.[5] Did you know? To date, there have been no confirmed deaths following an overdose of cannabis ingested for either recreational or medicinal purposes. Because of its effectiveness and relatively low incidence of side effects, cannabis is becoming increasingly popular as a treatment for a range of medical conditions, including arthritis, cancer, chronic pain, inflammatory bowel disease, depression, anxiety, fibromyalgia, insomnia, multiple sclerosis, Parkinson's disease, epilepsy, chemotherapy-related nausea, and post-traumatic stress disorder.[6]

Medical cannabis has been in use in various U.S. states starting in 1996, when California was the first to legalize it, and in Canada since it was legalized by the federal government in 2001. At that time, only around a hundred individuals signed on to the Health Canada program that would help them battle their chronic pain issues with cannabis. Today, over 300,000 Canadians and over 2 million Americans are registered as medical cannabis patients.[7] That might sound like a lot, but it isn't actually that high when we think about how many people suffering from chronic pain are still using various opioids extensively.

Even today, many health professionals are reluctant to prescribe medical cannabis to their patients due to a historical lack of information, education, or in-depth studies. Medically speaking, cannabis has also struggled to overcome the negative publicity of its popularity as a recreational drug. Many health professionals have tended to prescribe opioids instead in the belief that they will magically reduce pain with minimal side effects. However, as evidence has shown, the adverse effects of these drugs in cases of chronic pain are not to be taken lightly. Not only can their toxicity be fatal, but the physical dependency they create can render a state of deprivation in users and increase the risk of suicide. Opioids can be effective in the treatment of acute pain, but not chronic pain due to their potentially devastating long-term effects. In cases of chronic pain, a holistic approach to treatment is preferable in order to help patients retain their quality of life and functional ability.

In the past, medical cannabis would often be prescribed as a last resort, whereas today it is starting to be introduced to patients at an earlier stage, and even before certain opioid drugs. As it continues to be safely prescribed by the medical community and new studies are conducted, more specific therapeutic uses for medical cannabis are expected to emerge.

Could cannabis reduce overall opioid use by replacing opioid drugs in the treatment of chronic pain?[8] Let's take a closer look at this plant that has been used for centuries, if not millennia.

Recent studies have examined the physiological mechanisms of cannabis, helping to shed light on its effects on the body. The human body actually has its own endocannabinoid system, which produces chemical compounds that essentially give us the same kind of natural high as cannabis. To a greater or lesser extent, we all have these molecules in our bodies, as well as receptors in our brains that respond to our own endocannabinoids and any external cannabinoids we introduce to our bodies. The cannabinoid chemical compounds found in the brain and different parts of the body help to protect us and regulate our systems, entirely subconsciously. Could this be nature's way of equipping us with a remedy for the ailments of humanity?

When the body is unable to produce sufficient cannabinoids to protect itself against certain ailments, taking phytocannabinoids—cannabinoids that occur naturally in the cannabis plant—can help. Some people's systems are more sensitive to cannabinoids than others. Therefore, while a small dose may be more than enough for some people to feel the effects, it may take a far larger dose for others to experience a favorable response, and some may even experience an unfavorable response.

Scientific studies have tended to focus most extensively on two of the active components of cannabis: delta-9-tetrahydrocannabinol (THC) and cannabidiol (CBD). However, at least a hundred other cannabinoids can be found in different cannabis plants on which few, if any, studies have been conducted. In the years ahead, it will be interesting to see more of the benefits and drawbacks of this remarkable—and visually striking—plant come to light. It seems that the properties of cannabis may be even more beneficial than doctors and pain therapists originally thought.

When recreational cannabis was legalized in Canada in October of 2018, sales were so strong that stocks ran out in a matter of weeks. Demand has since continued to skyrocket. Meanwhile, prescriptions for medical cannabis continue to increase—perhaps a sign that more health professionals are broadening their horizons and looking into the therapeutic benefits.

I started to prescribe cannabis a number of years ago, somewhat tentatively because at the time it was out of the ordinary for doctors to do so, and studies were few and far between. Today, that is no longer the case as the benefits become more widely known and cannabis is increasingly seen as an effective natural drug for patients to try. Now there is no doubt that cannabis can reduce the excitability of pain receptors in the nervous system and can play a significant role in managing pain.[9] Just like any drug, however, cannabis may not be right for everyone. Similarly, it is important to tailor treatment and suitable doses to each individual patient.

Medical cannabis may be prescribed by doctors in Canada and the United States, as well as by nurse practitioners in Canada (except in Quebec, at least for now). Medical cannabis obtained on prescription from an authorized producer is no different from morphine sourced through a pharmacy; using it does not make you a criminal. Cannabis is a perfectly legal substance in all provinces and territories of Canada, as well as in many U.S. states that have embraced legalization. However, it's important to remember that it is prohibited to transport cannabis across international borders and many state lines. Users who attempt to enter another country or state with cannabis are likely to break the law and face serious criminal penalties. A medical prescription for cannabis is not a passport to travel to another country with it. In other words, Canadians are required to keep their cannabis in Canada, and Americans are advised to keep theirs within state lines, though the rules in some states may vary for medical marijuana patients. Before users consider leaving the country, they are advised to check the latest rules regarding the legality of their cannabis, legally prescribed or otherwise, as situations may change rapidly.

In Canada, the procedure for obtaining medical cannabis is straightforward. (Procedures in the United States vary by state.) Patients simply choose a Health Canada–licensed producer and submit an application form, which should take no more than a few minutes to complete. There is a short section for their authorized health practitioner to complete—as this is a medical document, it should specify the total quantity of THC prescribed. This will allow the practitioner to monitor the patient's therapeutic progress and gradually increase the dosage if need be. In my own practice, I typically prescribe a moderate dosage from the beginning (approximately 0.5 grams per day, as individuals in Canada are permitted to have up to 30 grams—just over an ounce—of dried marijuana in their possession in public). When patients come into my office for a follow-up consultation, I then adjust their prescription as required. Patients are typically free to determine the method of use that works best for them, as advised by their licensed producer's qualified technicians.

Cannabis obtained from a source other than a licensed producer remains illegal. What's more, street cannabis offers no guarantee of quality and, even more seriously, may contain toxins, pesticides, and other unknown additives. It is especially important to ensure that young adults using cannabis source a quality product, because the health of their growing brains ultimately depends on it. The legal age for cannabis consumption is eighteen in Alberta and nineteen in all other provinces and territories. In Quebec, where the legal age was originally eighteen, the limit has been raised to twenty-one. U.S. states where cannabis use is permitted have also tended to set the legal age at twenty-one.

All cannabis should be sourced from a licensed Health Canada facility (or in the United States, a state-licensed facility), as these producers are bound by strict quality standards. Because I make a point of checking the provenance of what I prescribe whenever possible, I paid a visit to one local licensed producer in Gatineau, Quebec. The first thing that struck me was the security gate on my way in. As well as having to provide my name, photo, and reasons for visiting the premises, I was assigned a guide by the producer to walk me through the facility. We had to don clean, white protective clothing—hat, masks, gloves, and all. Each area of the facility was locked and could only be accessed by the guide punching in a security code. I couldn't help but notice how clean everything was—even the walls, floors, and ceilings. It was also very warm inside the climate-controlled facility. I could smell the terpenes—the aromatic oils that give cannabis plants their distinctive scent and repel pests and predators. Some people find the smell of cannabis repulsive too—typically heady notes of skunk, lavender, sulfur, peppermint, and hops, though the odor can vary depending on the strain of cannabis as well as when it is dried and burned.

Not only was I struck by the cleanliness of the facility, I was also impressed by how environmentally minded it seemed. The glass roofs of the large greenhouses could slide open fully to let the warm summer air in, but surely a disadvantage of that would be exposing the plants to insects, I thought. And so, naturally, I asked the guide whether they had to use pesticides. I was assured that absolutely no insecticides or pesticides were used to control any bugs that found their way in. Instead, staff would identify the intruders and introduce appropriate predators, often ladybugs, to get rid of them. The idea was simple: introduce a few hungry ladybugs and let them feast on the intruding insects until they exhaust their own food supply and eventually die. The water used for the irrigation system is filtered and any surplus is collected and reused. To ensure maximum light exposure, a sophisticated lighting system is activated as soon as the slightest cloud floats overhead and casts a shadow on the plants. An entire team of specialized staff is also on hand to ensure optimal plant quality and health. Legal cannabis is subjected to a series of strict quality controls. There are no heavy metals, bacteria, or mold in a grow-op like this. The cannabis is then washed to eliminate any traces of fertilizer, and often sterilized by radiation. These procedures are particularly important for patients whose immune systems are compromised. Clearly, a pharmaceutical-quality product and an environmentally conscious production process are very important.

CBD AND THC

Of the 104 identified cannabinoids produced by the cannabis plant, the most commonly known are cannabidiol (CBD) and delta-9-tetrahydrocannabinol (THC), found in the leaves and flowering tops of the plant. The typical THC content of a plant is around 10 percent. Clearly, much remains to be discovered about other "new" cannabinoids and their therapeutic effects.

THC: Although THC is primarily known for its psychoactive properties and the euphoric high its users can experience, it also has powerful anti-inflammatory and pain-relieving effects. However, it may induce anxiety in some cases and be conducive to dependency for around 10 percent of users. It may even cause some users to experience psychotic episodes and hallucinations.

CBD: CBD is not addictive and has no psychoactive or euphoric effects, but it does have anti-inflammatory and mild pain-relieving properties, as well as being an effective antidepressant, anti-epileptic, anti-nausea, and anxiety-reducing agent. It can be an attractive option for patients as side effects are rare, other than some users reporting diarrhea, sedative effects, and changes in appetite. Strictly speaking, CBD should not be considered cannabis, since it only contains 0.2 percent THC. However, it should still be used with caution, since blood samples may still test positive for cannabis even if a person has only consumed CBD. Just like any drug, CBD may block certain hepatic enzymes and interact with other medication metabolized by the liver, so it's important that patients on daily medication consult with their doctor before taking CBD. Some patients may find that combining THC with CBD provides the pain relief they're looking for while minimizing the psychoactive effects of the THC. More studies will be needed to help determine the correct dosages and reveal all the benefits of these cannabinoids.

It's important to start gradually by consuming only small quantities of cannabis and choosing a strain with a higher concentration of CBD than THC before increasing the balance. Users are advised not to consume alcohol or other medication with cannabis, and rather than smoking it, to choose other methods of consuming cannabis. Patients should also avoid consuming cannabis too frequently and refrain from driving or working while impaired by cannabis. The consumption of cannabis may impair users' attention, memory, and learning capacity, and young people especially should be aware that regular use of cannabis before the age of twenty-five can interfere with the healthy development of their brains. If your interpersonal relationships are starting to suffer as a result of an excessive intake of cannabis, consider reducing your consumption. Anyone who feels that a family member of friend's behavior is suffering as a result of cannabis consumption would be wise to draw their attention to this gently and point out the dangers of excessive consumption and potential addiction. As with many other drugs and supplements, users should avoid consuming cannabis while pregnant and nursing, since no studies of the potential dangers have yet been carried out.

METHODS OF CONSUMPTION

Smoking. One method of consuming cannabis is to burn it in cigarette form and inhale the smoke. However, smoking is not considered to be a healthy method of consumption and is not recommended for individuals with respiratory disorders. Burning parts of the cannabis plant can actually release carcinogenic particles that can be up to five times more harmful to inhale than cigarette smoke.

It's more beneficial to inhale cannabis vapor using a **vaporizer** or **nebulizer**. These devices heat the cannabis to release its active components without generating any smoke. Cannabis has to go through a heat-driven process known as decarboxylation in order to activate its effects; as such, consuming the raw plant will have no effect, no matter how many leaves you munch.

Sublingual sprays offer another easy and practical method of delivery. Spraying a small quantity of decarboxylated cannabis oil—often mint-flavored—under the tongue is one of the faster and more subtle ways to deliver a dose of CBD or THC.

Capsules of decarboxylated (dried and activated) cannabis powder such as **HEXO Decarb** capsules are another popular method of consumption, with only one to three capsules typically required to produce the desired effect. Some people find this method easier and more socially acceptable, since it's just like popping a pill.

Ingesting cannabis in edible form is an easy and slow-acting way to experience the effects of cannabis. Compared to smoking, ingesting edibles takes longer to produce the desired effect—typically over an hour—but the effects are also more long-lasting, sometimes for up to eight hours. Because the cannabinoids are slower to take effect, users may find they need to need to ingest twice the quantity to feel the effects. Cannabis can easily be incorporated into baked goods such as muffins, cookies, brownies, and even croissants, and edible cannabis is also readily available in the form of gummy candies, juice, and other beverages.

Cannabis-infused skin creams are another interesting option, because they allow patients to treat specific parts of the body without feeling the effects of cannabis throughout their entire system.

A while ago, a patient of mine—let's call her Sylvia—consulted with me for fibromyalgia. She was a dynamic fifty-two-year-old entrepreneur who had been suffering from chronic pain issues since she turned twenty. Over the years, she had undergone a lot of tests, tried a lot of remedies, and made changes to her lifestyle, as well as taking anti-inflammatories and opioid painkillers. She came to me to try a different drug-based approach because she was suffering from drowsiness, memory problems, and constipation on her existing prescription medication.

To her great surprise, I suggested she try cannabis. "Is it legal, and is it right for someone like me?" she asked. I recommended a sublingual medical cannabis spray with CBD oil, together with a CBD and THC cream for her to apply to the painful areas. She was astounded to see a substantial reduction of her pain. Not only that, her sleep improved and the constipation went away. Her mother, who was suffering from insomnia and osteoarthritis pain in her shoulder, saw the improvement in her daughter's condition and how much better she was sleeping, and decided to sneak a try of her peppermint-flavored aerosol spray. Sylvia had only told her mother that she was taking a natural remedy for her condition, because cannabis was still very much a taboo at the time. She didn't want her mother to know she was "using pot," worried that a woman of her age—seventy-eight—would be mortified by the thought. Sylvia's mother then decided to try some of her daughter's cream for her shoulder pain. A few days later, she innocently admitted that she had found a very effective cream for her osteoarthritis on Sylvia's nightstand. It took a few weeks before Sylvia plucked up the courage to tell her mother that her "natural remedies" contained cannabis. Her mother's jaw dropped, before she quickly composed herself and quipped that she always knew nature's pharmacy did things best.

Stay active, stay healthy

I can't stress the importance of exercise enough. It will change your life for the better. As well as helping to reduce pain, exercise allows you to simply get more out of life. Exercise in itself is beneficial and it will always play a preventive role when it comes to health.

Have you ever noticed how animated and full of life children are? They dance, twirl, and run so much, it can be dizzying. Movement is life, while inertia breeds sickness, atrophy, and destruction. Movement stimulates blood flow throughout the body, delivering fuel and displacing toxins—essentially the body's garbage.

There's no doubt about it: we were made to move. But for many of us as adults, the muscle in our body that always seems to get the hardest workout is our brain. We bombard our brains with a constant stream of thoughts that go beyond the bounds of mental exercise and threaten to wear us out completely. We need to flex more than just our mental muscles if we want to keep stiffness at bay, avoid weight problems, and ward off the plethora of inflammatory conditions to which we humans are susceptible; the body is a marvelous machine, but it's also demanding. Fortunately, by moving our bodies, we will consistently improve our circulation and mobility. The more we move, the deeper good health takes root.

Not so long ago, when a patient suffered a heart attack, doctors would prescribe rest and a complete lack of physical activity out of fear of recurrence. Today, however, we promote exercise to encourage rehabilitation and reduce the risk of relapse. Physical inactivity reduces cardiac contraction and vascularization, promotes arterial hypertension, and increases stress and anxiety—as well as pain. Just because we're experiencing pain, it doesn't mean we should stop moving or doing exercise. Following an exercise program can promote circulation, reduce pain, and accelerate a return to health.

In seniors, more hip fractures are due to a lack of exercise than a lack of calcium. And many older people are too quick to rely on a walker to get around. This leads to rapid degeneration of muscle mass and hinders balance, so that down the line, even the slightest movement can cause the person to lose their balance and be unable to break their fall and get up again properly. I can never emphasize too much how important physical exercise is for this segment of the population—especially for those in seniors' homes. It's not just a question of being in shape; it's essential for our health in general.

RESUMING EXERCISE
AFTER AN INJURY

If you've suffered an injury, it's crucial to think about how you'll resume exercise. Physical rehabilitation—the branch of medicine that guides recovery following illness, accident, or injury—plays a crucial role in restoring the patient's mobility, helping them recover as much functional capacity as possible while reducing their pain and improving their quality of life. Working with a professional to re-educate your body can help you not only regain mobility more quickly, but also sidestep some serious postural issues. I would advise consulting a specialist, since every treatment should be personalized to minimize pain and avoid the risk of lasting disability. If you're experiencing pain following a muscle or joint injury, nerve damage, or cardio-respiratory issues, a rehabilitation specialist will be able to guide you through the techniques involved in recovering optimal function.

So you don't have time to go to the gym three times a week, and you don't feel like taking fitness classes you think are too expensive or too much hard work? Not to mention the pain that's confining you to your bed or your armchair? It's easy to make excuses, but it is worth persevering. Even modest activity will be beneficial for your physical health and your morale.

Obviously, if you're in pain, be careful, because pain is a warning light that shouldn't be ignored. However, some mild exercise in moderation will usually be beneficial. Individuals with fibromyalgia should have an exercise program tailored to their needs—otherwise sedentariness may aggravate their condition.

Here are a few tips that will make a difference for your health without leaving a dent in your wallet or your busy schedule. You can put these into practice every day. Exercise shouldn't feel like a chore, though, so don't feel guilty if you're not very active one day—maybe you feel too lethargic, or you don't have time because you had to stay late at work. You might find it easier to do more exercise on your days off. Either way, since you need to be active, you might as well be enthusiastic about it!

STEP IT UP

Do your legs feel heavy? Do you experience frequent cramps, back pain, stiff knees, or shortness of breath? Well, try taking a brisk walk. When you're out and about, try leaving your car a little farther away from your destination. It'll probably be easier to find a parking space, and it will give you a chance to walk and breathe a little before you get where you're going. If you're headed to work, be mindful of your walk and take the time to breathe and make the most of this time to yourself. Put a spring in your step and enjoy the lightness of the day ahead.

TAKE THE STAIRWAY TO HEALTH

Have you given up on those step classes at the gym? Don't worry, there's no exercise police waiting to give you a ticket. Did you know you can do step for free? Simply take the stairs as often as you can to build a strong heart. Cardiologists everywhere are prescribing this simple exercise that will flex your cardiac muscles, tone up your lower limbs, and even strengthen your bones!

USE PEDAL POWER TO STAY A STEP AHEAD

If you own a bike, you're lucky to be able to spin a little more discipline into your exercise program. Take a little time to turn the pedals, and your heart and whole body will thank you. You'll even give your immune system a boost, so you won't be as vulnerable to any bugs that are going around. Now that hybrid electric bikes are becoming more common, it's easier than ever to go that extra mile and breeze your way up the hills, or simply take it easy on two wheels if you're not feeling very energetic—no more excuses for not getting out there! E-bikes are good at giving your health as well as your speed a boost, so long as you put in some effort. (If you don't pedal at all, you're not going to get very far.)

TONE UP WITH STRENGTH TRAINING

The older you get, the more your muscle mass loses its tone. You'll find the natural pull of gravity keeps getting stronger, too. To stay in shape, you'll have to increase your protein intake and cut down on sugar. It's also a good idea to do some strength training with light weights or resistance bands to boost your muscle mass. Your body will thank you! People with reduced mobility would be wise to seek professional guidance to avoid aggravating their muscles and joints.

RUN TO REDUCE STRESS

A friend of mine once asked me why I suggested he should take up running. I told him it was one of the most natural ways for us to stay in shape. "Well, it doesn't come naturally to me," he joked.

Nature is a timeless source of wisdom, life, and beauty, and I draw a lot of inspiration from it in my practice. If you don't always have time to go to the gym or feel like exercising, you're not alone. About ten years ago, I found myself wondering how animals in their natural habitat managed to stay healthy and in good shape. After all, obesity and sickness are very rare beasts in the animal kingdom. I wondered what makes it so easy for animals to keep in shape, since they don't have gym memberships or keep a set of weights in the grass ready to pump iron. There are no bikes for them to ride in the wild, no stairs for them to climb, and no nutritionists to keep them trim on a special diet. So, what do they know that we don't know?

Imagine for a moment that you're a zebra on the savanna. You're grazing on the grass without a care in the world, slowly making your way to a pond for a little refreshment. All is calm beneath the blazing sun. Just as you're craning your neck out over the water to take a drink, your ears prick up. There's a rustling coming from the tall grass, and that's not good news. You turn around just in time to see the shadow of a lion ready to pounce and sink its claws into you. In a flash, you take to your heels and gallop off as fast as you can, trying to put as much distance as possible between yourself and your ravenous predator. For the next minute or so, you run for your life, leaving the hunter in the dust, forced to give up the chase.

Like many animals, the zebra only exercises appreciably and to the point of exhaustion when its survival is at stake. When the time comes for it to run for its life, it gives its all for a short burst, and that's typically the only intensive exercise it gets for the next three to five days. Running is a healthy exercise that's perfectly natural for most animals—and it used to be for humans too, before we invented weapons. It has always been in our nature to run.

Let's take a closer look at what happened when you were a zebra being chased. You went through an intensely stressful experience, albeit very short-lived, as your fight-or-flight response was triggered. By way of comparison, many of us humans "run" around all day under constant stress. This overstimulates the sympathetic nervous system and is akin to keeping a finger on the fight-or-flight response trigger. It's been proved: stress is slowly killing us, because it's inflammatory. How then can we survive in a world of chronic tension and anxiety? By reducing stress, practicing relaxation, and doing exercise. Intense exercise is ideal, because it quickly burns off adrenaline and cortisol, the stress hormone secreted by the adrenal glands. In short: whenever you're under a lot of stress, try going for a quick sprint (or do another kind of strenuous exercise) that will get you out of breath. We have Mother Nature to thank for making this such a practical, afford-able, and pleasant lesson to learn.

TABATA: GO FOR IT!

Science has recently suggested that one of the healthiest things for us is intense bursts of exercise, such as short, fast sprints. Enter the Tabata method—twenty seconds of hard effort, followed by ten seconds of rest, repeated for four minutes. Pioneered by Dr. Izumi Tabata, this approach has the power to increase cardio-respiratory capacity more than an hour of moderate exercise.[10] Try it and you'll see: stand up and run on the spot as fast as you can for twenty seconds. Now pause for ten seconds, take a few deep breaths, and repeat until four minutes have gone by. That's it—you're done! I just did the same thing before writing these words, and believe me, it's a stimulation for all the senses. Variable-intensity interval running is now my main form of exercise. Several times a week, I run hard for thirty seconds or a minute at a time, then I walk for a minute. I repeat the same sequence three more times, and that's my workout—I feel great even after such a short burst of exercise. However, I'd advise doing a few stretches first to avoid pulling a muscle. I also suggest doing some light stretching after exercising to promote a return to normal muscle tone and prevent any painful contractions from occurring during the rest phase.

STRENGTH EXERCISES TO RELAX YOUR NECK AND SHOULDERS

If you've been reading this book for a while, or even sitting at your computer for a few minutes, it's probably time you relaxed your neck and shoulders. Here are some super-simple exercises that will both strengthen and relax the muscles around your neck and shoulder blades.

Isometric exercises involve contracting a muscle or group of muscles tightly without any actual movement. The idea here is to contract the muscles while the hands hold the head straight and steady. Do the contractions in every direction (forward, backward, to the left, and to the right) without moving your head or neck. As you breathe in, hold the contraction for seven seconds, using your hands to stop your head from moving. As you breathe out, relax your shoulders and let your arms hang down at your sides. Do this two or three times. You'll soon feel your muscles relax and even notice improved blood flow to your neck and head.

Go on: step away from the computer, or put the book down, and place your hands in the position you see in the illustrations. It's very important to keep your head still by resisting the pressure exerted by your hands.

Isometric exercises to relieve neck stiffness

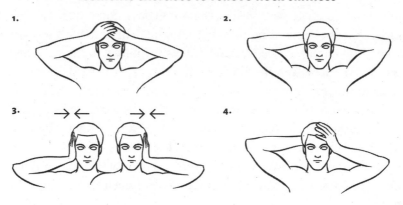

The two isometric exercises below will help release shoulder tension by relaxing the muscles as well as increasing muscle tone and strength and improving circulation to this area.

Isometric exercises to relieve shoulder tension

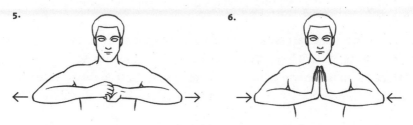

YOGA EXERCISES TO PROTECT YOUR JOINTS

For many years, I have done five minutes of yoga exercises every morning after my shower. It's not a lot of time, but it's enough to stay flexible, which is so important for our joints, tendons, and ligaments, as well as for stimulating circulation. I have recommended these exercises to many patients (with variations depending on their age) to great success.

EXERCISE ROUTINE FOR THE SPINE

These exercises will promote proper spinal function and relax the spinal musculature. Do them slowly, using as little energy as possible. These movements shouldn't hurt. If you find some painful, skip them and try them again another time.

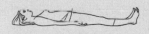

Corpse pose: Lie on your back with your arms by your sides and take long, slow breaths through your nose. Clear your mind and allow your muscles to relax.

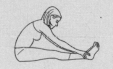

Seated forward fold: Start in a seated position with your legs straight out in front of you. Lean forward and try to touch your toes.

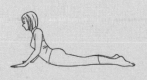

Cobra: Lie on your stomach with your hands under your shoulders, pressing your pelvis down on the ground, and push gently into your hands to extend your spine. Start by keeping your arms bent a little. After a few sessions, you can work toward extending them fully.

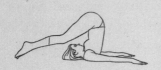

Plow pose: Lie on your back and slowly raise your legs over your head. This allows your spine to bend deeply and brings maximum blood flow to the brain.

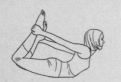

Bow pose: Lie on your stomach and reach for your ankles with your hands. Straighten your arms as you kick your feet away from you, and enjoy the spinal extension.

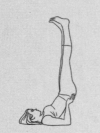

Shoulder stand: Lie on your back and press your legs tightly together. Roll back onto your shoulder blades and lift your legs into the air, using your hands to support your pelvis. Keep your legs as straight as you can and try to push the soles of your feet toward the ceiling. This exercise improves circulation to the spine and internal organs.

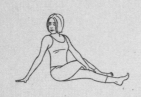

Seated spinal twist: Do this exercise to stretch both sides of your spine and torso. Start in a seated position with straight legs. Bend your right knee and move your right foot to the other side of your left leg. Reach your left hand over your bent right leg to touch your left knee (this helps to hold your pelvis steady). Then, keeping your back straight, rotate your torso to the right (you may hear a cracking sound). Slowly return to center and repeat on the other side.

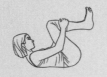

Knees to chest pose: Lie on your back and hug your knees into your chest. Gently roll back and forth to give your spine a little massage.

Detoxify now

Detoxification is the process of eliminating toxins and waste products from the body. The human body is constantly detoxifying itself. Filtration happens in the liver and kidneys, while elimination occurs through perspiration and the passing of stools. Patients often ask me about the best way to detox their bodies and are keen to consume all kinds of supplements. Perhaps the most effective detoxifier, however, is good old-fashioned exercise. Exercise can have a powerful detoxifying effect by improving overall circulation to not only the muscles but also the liver, kidneys, and intestines. During exercise, the heart pumps blood to the organs faster, which helps to eliminate toxins more quickly and at a deeper level. Exercise also improves essential circulatory functions such as venous and lymphatic return. Add sweat to the mix and the body's largest organ—the skin—gets a workout eliminating toxins too.

FAR INFRARED SAUNAS

If you can afford it, investing in a far infrared sauna is a wonderful way to give your body a general detox on a regular basis.

Unlike traditional saunas, which warm the body by heating the air with stones on a wood-fired or electric stove, far infrared saunas deep-heat the body with infrared radiation that is invisible to the human eye. While early models of these saunas used ceramic elements to heat the air and emit the beneficial far infrared radiation, more recent saunas are now using carbon fiber heaters, which perform better and are more energy-efficient.

One of the benefits of far infrared saunas is that compared to traditional saunas, lower temperatures are required to obtain the desired effect: 120 to 140 degrees Fahrenheit as opposed to around 210 degrees Fahrenheit. Also, they heat the body directly, not just the air. Infrared heat can penetrate up to two inches beneath the skin, providing a faster, more efficient, and arguably more pleasant experience than traditional saunas. As sweat is released through the skin, it carries toxins and heavy metals, such as aluminum, lead, and mercury, out of the body. This helps get rid of the various contaminants we're exposed to through the air we breathe and the water we drink.[11] A few thousand dollars will buy you a compact far infrared sauna that can accommodate two to four people.

When the twin towers of the World Trade Center in New York fell on 9/11, the efforts of firefighters and other rescuers were severely hampered by the heat, dust, and smoke from the giant inferno and poisonous air; many of these first responders have ended up suffering severe long-term health effects as a result. A physician colleague in the United States told me about how some of the rescuers who were urgently hospitalized were given infrared sauna treatments for several hours a day for several weeks, combined with niacin (vitamin B) supplements to improve blood circulation at the skin level. The profound sweating induced by the infrared helped these patients to eliminate many kinds of toxins and heavy metals they ingested at Ground Zero. During the sauna treatment, their sweat would turn the hospital towels blue—likely a sign of elimination of manganese, a toxic metal.

WEIGHING IN ON MERCURY AND LEAD

While we're on the subject of detoxification, let's broach a more controversial topic. Is the mercury in dental amalgams harmful to health? It's a debate that has divided dentists' opinions for years. One thing's for sure: lead and mercury are heavy metals and neurotoxins. To reduce toxic lead pollution in the air, paint no longer contains this heavy metal as an ingredient and the gasoline we put in our vehicles is now unleaded. Years ago, dental amalgams used to contain a lot of lead, until bans on this ingredient were gradually implemented by the health authorities. But what about the mercury in today's gray dental fillings—isn't that toxic too?

When dentists place an amalgam filling, they wear a mask and gloves and even use a powerful vacuum pump to remove the mercury vapors. Every year, dentists around the world fill our mouths with hundreds of tons of mercury. By way of example, France alone uses seventeen tons of the stuff per year in composite dental amalgams, which contain 50 percent mercury.[12]

When I was a child, I was fascinated by this curious silver liquid. I remember that one day I had fun playing with a broken old thermometer, marveling at the fine droplets of mercury that wouldn't stick to the floor but amalgamated when I pushed them together. Only years later did I realize how dangerous that was.

These days we've stopped filling thermometers with mercury, but we keep filling our mouths with the stuff when we get a cavity treated at the dentist's office. I find this very curious. There are international agreements to reduce mercury emissions around the world. Eliminating this toxic waste from the environment is a global problem, as we struggle to find ways to dispose of such a persistent pollutant. Since 2002, dental facilities have been required to use amalgam separators to recover waste material safely and prevent it from leaching into the groundwater table. If it's not legal anymore to flush these amalgams down the toilet bowl, are our mouths really a safe environment for the stuff?

Certainly, in dental fillings, mercury is used in its solid form, and many dentists maintain that it's inert and won't leach into other parts of the body when it's in place in the tooth. Leading toxicology experts have also assured us that no one has died from mercury poisoning since amalgams were first introduced in the early 1800s. However, by 1840, the American Society of Dental Surgeons deemed amalgams to be dangerous and ordered its members to stop using them. It was only in 1859, however, when advocates for mercury formed their own association (since renamed the American Dental Association), that amalgams reappeared in America.

According to some toxicologists, dental mercury is both carcinogenic and mutagenic, and therefore toxic for the nervous, immune, and hormone systems. Mercury can accumulate anywhere in the body and is hard to eliminate. It particularly affects the brain and can even cross the placenta and contaminate breast milk.[13]

Health Canada has placed mercury on a list of "toxic materials targeted for eventual elimination," and acknowledges that having at least four amalgams causes mercury to be released into the body in amounts exceeding the permitted daily intake level.[14] According to Health Canada, "Dentists are to be encouraged to decrease the use of amalgam and other restorative materials through the use of diagnostic and preventive treatment strategies based on tooth structure preservation." For the moment, you can ask your dentist to explore alternative options to amalgams.

In 2013, a new convention on mercury was adopted by 140 countries with a view to reducing its use by encouraging dentists to change their practices and use composite or ceramic materials instead. Norway, Sweden, and Denmark have outlawed mercury from all new dental fillings.

Could mercury be to blame for chronic illness? Is there a link between mercury and neurodegenerative diseases, such as Parkinson's, dementia, Alzheimer's, and multiple sclerosis, or immune disorders? The questions remain unanswered. As we rely on the relevant authorities to give the issue serious consideration, many associations are calling for mercury to be banned immediately, given the ready availability of far less toxic alternatives. Another word of caution, however: removing fillings is not something to be taken lightly. All interventions on an existing amalgam filling are subject to a very strict safety protocol.[15]

I distinctly recall one patient about twenty years ago who had a number of dental amalgams. She was a teacher who took a very proactive approach to her health and led an exemplary lifestyle, eating a balanced diet and getting plenty of exercise and relaxation. One day, she decided to get all her fillings removed, because she was concerned about the possible dangers of dental mercury. She was in such a hurry to have the offending matter taken out, she went to see a dentist right away and only came to me two months later, when she was suffering from unexplained fatigue, emotional instability, and difficulty concentrating. She had always been active and healthy, and now she was so exhausted she had to take time off work.

Her blood work came back perfectly normal, and nothing seemed out of the ordinary when I examined her. As I was telling her I couldn't find anything medically wrong with her, I had a brain wave and asked whether her dentist had taken all the right precautions for such a mass extraction. I figured that performing such a major procedure without a strict protocol and the proper follow-up might have resulted in mercury poisoning by inhalation. As it turned out, no such protocol had been followed in her case. The patient's symptoms persisted for nearly a year in spite of multiple treatments.

Because mercury isn't harmless for everyone, it's important to talk to your dentist before rushing into anything, especially as some have specialized knowledge about dental mercury. Dentists (who work with mercury, obviously) are three times more likely than the average person to suffer memory issues and depression and ten times more likely to contract renal diseases[16] probably because of handling mercury.

About fifteen years ago, I was attending a three-day training in the United States with Dr. Dietrich Klinghardt, a German specialist who was there to demonstrate a variety of techniques for relieving pain. On the second day, a former dentist and professor at the University of Calgary School of Medicine, Dr. Murray Vimy, came to talk to us about a research project he had carried out some years earlier about dental amalgams. I was curious as to what the connection with chronic pain could be, and why he was there to give a talk about fillings. He explained his concern about the danger of mercury poisoning in the body.

Dr. Vimy placed amalgam fillings in around thirty sheep to observe what mercury would do to their bodies. Why sheep? In humans, it's not uncommon for mercury amalgams to stay in the mouth for twenty years, but sheep are ruminants and are constantly grinding their teeth. This enabled Dr. Vimy to conduct the study in a matter of months rather than years. He decided to run the study over six months and had the brilliant idea of using mercury with radioactive isotopes so that the mercury could be traced by radiological methods.

To his great surprise, after just a few days, he could see the radioactive mercury isotopes emerging from the edges of the teeth and entering the gum tissue. The more time went by, the more the mercury seeped its way into various organs, including the brain, liver, heart, and kidneys. These observations were astounding. Worse still, one of the ewes was pregnant, and her fetus was soon glowing with radiation in its brain and many of its other organs, which meant that the mercury had crossed the placental membrane. Believing he had finally established a connection between systemic mercury and dental amalgams, he presented his findings at a major international dental conference.[17] Imagine his surprise when his arguments were dismissed on the pretext that humans were not sheep and didn't grind their teeth as much. Obviously, Dr. Vimy knew very well that humans aren't ruminants, but given how short his study had been, he was still convinced it spoke volumes.

Determined to make his point, he conducted a further study, this time on monkeys. Unlike sheep, they eat a varied diet, have teeth similar to ours, and do not spend all day ruminating. This time, he conducted the experiment over a slightly longer period of time— about a year—and found the same results. And so, he went before a committee again to present the findings of his research, only to have his radiological techniques discredited on the basis that the restorative material used in humans would be somewhat different. Make of this what you will...

DAY AFTER DAY, we go about most of our regular activities so quickly and subconsciously we often barely realize what we're doing, whether it's getting out of bed, brushing our teeth, washing our hair, pulling on our socks and shoes, eating, or swatting a fly away from our nose. To turn the page on this chapter, I'd like to suggest we put our ADLS—activities of daily living—on a "diet." Let's try abstaining from doing things too quickly, unconsciously, or out of habit, only to forget what we've done barely two minutes later, being so lost in our thoughts.

There's a simple exercise that can help us all be more mindful of our everyday actions. All we have to do is take our time. When we do anything more slowly, we do it more mindfully. This goes for everything we do in life. Even if we slow down by just 30 percent, we will be more present.

It's time we brought more presence to our daily routines. Let's embrace this new habit and channel our energy to experience a calmer, happier, and more fulfilled life and enjoy greater peace of mind and body.

Remember to turn the page slowly and be fully present when you start reading the next chapter!

CHAPTER 6

Ways to Treat Pain

|||||||||||||||||||||||||||||||||||||||||||||||||||||||||

HOPE: Hold On, Pain Ends

ANON

T HERE ARE PLENTY of treatment options for overcoming pain, and different approaches may be called for depending on the severity, immediacy, and chronicity of the pain. Some are basic and easy to implement even at home, as we saw in the last chapter, while others must be administered by health professionals. This chapter can serve as a guide, but it's not a replacement for a professional medical opinion or diagnosis regarding the cause of the pain.

Pain medications

||||||||||||||||||||||||||||||||||||||||||||||||||

I've always been of the opinion that Eastern and Western medicine are complementary. That's why I see no contradiction in the fact that I practice acupuncture and Western medicine side by side, depending on the circumstances. This includes prescribing medication, when necessary.

It's worth bearing in mind that medicine in the Western world has its distant origins in shamanic healing, which often used tree barks and plants. Aspirin was originally derived from willow bark, for instance, while morphine traces its origins to the opium poppy. Many drugs are rooted in nature and were created by modifying natural chemical compounds, adding certain substances to make synthetic analgesics that could be patented to ensure profits for the pharmaceutical companies. While there's no shortage of painkillers on the market, there are currently no drugs that can make chronic pain go away. In other words, no medicine can completely eradicate pain. When you contract an infection, your physician can prescribe an antibiotic or antiseptic, and you'll get completely better. Painkillers, however, only have a temporary effect.

While aspirin, non-steroidal anti-inflammatory drugs (NSAIDs), morphine, opiates, and their derivatives (such as codeine) are typically prescribed for pain relief, physicians have also started prescribing other drugs with different therapeutic indications that were found to have pain-relieving properties as an additional effect. We still know very little about how the brain will function under the effect of any drug, and it's often only by chance that we discover how an epilepsy drug, for instance, can also relieve pain.

Increasingly, antidepressants are being prescribed for pain, especially to treat fibromyalgia. Tricyclic antidepressants such as Elavil are one example, as are some newer antidepressants such as Cipralex. These are referred to as **symptomatic drugs**, because they only treat the symptoms, not the cause.

How do these antidepressants relieve pain? Under the effect of a greater concentration of certain neurotransmitters (page 37), the brain likely feels less pain, or feels it differently. This doesn't eliminate the source of the pain, but patients feel some relief. However, Elavil can cause numbness and lead to drowsiness in certain individuals.

Other drugs frequently prescribed for pain include antiepileptics such as gabapentin (Neurontin) and pregabalin (Lyrica). These drugs, initially developed for epilepsy, were found to also be effective against pain by modifying the pain signal and blocking the formation of neurotransmitters.

AN IMPORTANT TIP FOR TAKING MEDICATION

When you're prescribed pain medication, the goal of the treatment is to relieve the pain, and it's crucial to follow the prescribed dosage. Recovery is dependent on the patient being able to relax because the medication reduces their pain. Too often, though, I've seen patients wait until their pain gets very bad before taking their medication, because they say they don't want to become dependent. This approach can make it difficult to accurately assess the extent of the pain and can ultimately lead the patient to require an increased drug dosage, hindering recovery.

If you take a dosage as prescribed and the pain reappears or increases before the time comes to take the next dose, this means that the current treatment is insufficient and will require a revised dosage in order to bring relief.

Another common issue is that some patients are reluctant to take their medication because they're worried that they won't know if their condition worsens if they can't feel the pain. Most often, in fact, the opposite tends to happen. Because the medication is intended to provide temporary relief, if the pain increases, you'll notice it, and the physician will generally try to find out why. In cases like these, relieving the pain can help us to treat it more effectively.

To be effective, painkillers must be taken at specific times of day, even if the pain hasn't reappeared. This ensures a continuous pain-relieving action and allows for additional doses (interdoses) if required to relieve spikes in pain that may occur despite regular treatment. When treating constant pain, doctors will often prescribe a continuous slow-release drug. This can streamline treatment to one dose per day and can often help the patient avoid unpleasant side effects, since the drug is released more slowly.

A growing number of drugs are now available as transdermal patches—including **fentanyl**, a morphine derivative developed in

Belgium in the 1950s. Fentanyl has recently garnered a somewhat controversial reputation due to its use as a street drug and the high risk of fatal overdose it presents, especially when administered orally or intravenously. Due to misuse it has become one of the most deadly drugs currently on the market. In 2017, there were more than 47,000 apparent opioid-related deaths in the United States; opioid overdoses kill more Americans than gun violence or car accidents. In Canada the same year, there were over 4,000 deaths, 72 percent of which involved fentanyl.[1] These numbers have continued to rise by around 40 percent annually.

WHY IS FENTANYL SO DANGEROUS?

Fentanyl is one of the most powerful synthetic opioid painkillers ever produced. It is thirty times more potent than heroin and a hundred times more potent than morphine. This means that it does not take a large quantity to cause a potentially fatal overdose.

When fentanyl is used under proper medical direction and supervision, it can be very effective at treating intense and cancer-related pain. It is typically administered as a transdermal patch for patients to change every seventy-two hours, orally in tablet form, or by injection in hospitals. When the drug is administered transdermally, a safe dosage is released slowly and gradually into the patient's bloodstream, providing relief from pain and a euphoric, relaxing effect. However, like all opioids, it affects the respiratory system; if too high a dose is administered, it will lead to respiratory depression and potentially cause the patient to stop breathing. Fentanyl travels far more quickly than heroin to the part of the brain that controls breathing, so an individual may very suddenly find themselves struggling or unable to breathe. Many people who overdose are simply unaware of the potency of the drug and do not suspect that such a small dose can be so dangerous.

Fentanyl can enter the illegal drug market by way of theft of pharmaceutical fentanyl products, illegal import from other countries, or production by clandestine laboratories.[2] There is always the danger that any illegal street drug may contain fentanyl in any quantity, and even a few grains can be fatal. Fentanyl is odorless and tasteless, so it can easily go undetected by unsuspecting users. Health Canada offers drug-checking services and fentanyl test strips through supervised drug consumption sites, which can help users detect traces of fentanyl in illegal drugs. (In the United States, these strips are increasingly available through overdose-prevention groups and public-health organizations in some states and cities.)

The signs of a fentanyl or other opioid overdose include sleepiness, slow and shallow breathing, blue lips, cold and clammy skin, and tiny pupils. If you think someone is overdosing on fentanyl or any other opioid, you should call 911 immediately, try to help the person to keep breathing, and, if available, use naloxone, a drug that can temporarily reverse the effects. Regardless of whether it is administered intravenously, orally, through mucous membranes, or through the skin, fentanyl poses a high risk for illegal drug users. The safest way for this extremely potent drug to be administered is as a slow-release patch under proper medical supervision.

ACETYLSALICYLIC ACID

Acetylsalicylic acid (ASA; aspirin) is an analgesic (painkiller), anti-inflammatory, and antipyretic (fever-reducing) drug all rolled into one. It also acts as a blood thinner and can reduce blood clotting, so it's often recommended in very small doses (81 mg) as a preventive treatment for heart disease and stroke patients. ASA can have undesirable side effects, such as heartburn and gastric issues ranging in severity from irritation to ulcerations of the gastric wall. Those with sensitivities should therefore avoid aspirin, even in small doses. In all cases, it's important to take this medication as prescribed.

NON-STEROIDAL ANTI-INFLAMMATORY DRUGS (NSAIDS)

Other anti-inflammatories include non-steroidal anti-inflammatory drugs (NSAIDS), perhaps most notably ibuprofen (Advil, Motrin). NSAIDS can be taken in conjunction with acetaminophen (Tylenol). While many NSAIDS are available over the counter, some are available only by prescription. As all NSAIDS can cause gastric irritation and increased vascular risk, it's advisable to take them with food.

The number of new NSAIDS on the market seems to have exploded in the last twenty years or so—excessively so, in my opinion. Often, these new molecular formulas work in very similar ways, and marketing hype is what propels them to bestselling-drug status. Some big-name drugs have even been taken off the market due to their toxic effect on the blood vessels. This was the case with Vioxx, for example, which was found to have caused thousands of heart attacks and deaths, as mentioned in Chapter 3. We should be mindful of the risks of buying into the marketing hype surrounding new drugs on the market, for which the public may end up bearing the cost.

ACUTE INFLAMMATION: THE GATEWAY TO HEALING

In any acute inflammatory process, various proteins in the body are altered—specifically collagen, the supportive tissue that makes up 30 percent of the total protein in the body. An acute inflammatory reaction is short-lived, essentially sounding the alarm to set the repair-and-regenerate process in motion and restore the area to its former state of stability. Acute inflammation therefore has an important role to play, because it tells the body to wake up and repair the damage ASAP.

The key thing to remember is that it isn't necessarily a good idea to reduce acute inflammation initially, because that reaction warns the body that something is wrong and needs repair.

In the initial hours following a trauma, a mild anti-inflammatory painkiller is ideal for taking the edge off the inflammation. On another note, if you're going into surgery, it's generally advisable to stop taking any cortisone-based anti-inflammatory medication a few days before to ensure it doesn't interfere with the body's natural inflammatory process post-surgery, which is important for a speedy recovery.

Acute inflammation is a biological necessity, and it's a perfectly healthy part of any trauma or illness. Treating acute inflammation with an anti-inflammatory won't remedy the cause; it will only alleviate a symptom and may even compromise the healing process. The current vision of modern medicine—with its tendency to treat ailments with symptomatic drugs—contradicts the principles of functional medicine and other more natural, preventive approaches, which seek first and foremost to correct the underlying causes of the imbalances in the body we have labeled as illness.

By contrast, my approach shifts the focus to guiding and stimulating the different facets of self-regulation and healing. As I pointed out earlier, we should be treating the initial source of the problem while also helping the body to build up its own capacity to respond positively to the attacks and imbalances it encounters.

ACETAMINOPHEN

Acetaminophen (Tylenol, Atasol) acts solely as an analgesic and doesn't generally cause any gastric issues. However, to avoid the risk of severe liver damage, it's important not to exceed the recommended dose.

TRAMADOL

Another painkiller, tramadol, has been well known in Europe for over twenty years. Similar to codeine, this moderate-strength analgesic is generally well tolerated. Interestingly, the tramadol molecule has a mild narcotic effect and works through interfering with pain-signal transmission in the brain. What's more, tramadol releases two neurotransmitters, norepinephrine and serotonin, which also reduce pain and positively affect mood.

ANTIDEPRESSANTS

Antidepressants are generally effective at relieving pain and have the advantage of not creating dependency. However, it's important to bear in mind that addiction can be psychological as well as physical.

ANTICONVULSANTS

These drugs were initially developed to treat epilepsy, and their pain-relieving properties were only discovered later. Commonly prescribed today, the main drugs in this category are carbamazepine (Tegretol), gabapentin (Neurontin), and pregabalin (Lyrica). Side effects may include drowsiness, dizziness, and nausea.

NARCOTICS

Morphine-like medications are derived from opium. Contrary to popular belief, they aren't necessarily dangerous or too powerful, and their prescription isn't necessarily an indicator of the intensity of the illness—if your doctor prescribes narcotic-based medication, it doesn't necessarily mean your condition is severe. These drugs have been on the market for a very long time and, in small doses in the short term, they present very few side effects, the most frequent being constipation, nausea, and sedation.

As the strength of narcotics is consistent with their weight, the potency of a given drug can be measured in milligrams, though the potency of two different drugs with the same milligram value won't necessarily be comparable. (For example, 30 mg of codeine is less potent than just 15 mg of morphine.) These drugs are particularly beneficial after operations; when prescribed intravenously, they are potent and fast-acting, though this is when their side effects tend to be greater, especially on top of the aftereffects of surgery and anesthesia. In tablet form at a low dose of 5 mg, a narcotic is unlikely to have any unpleasant effects. Higher doses of 60 mg or more may be administered depending on the circumstances.

The danger of narcotics lies in the potential for addiction. Even so, addiction is not as frequent an occurrence as it was once thought to be, and not every patient will be susceptible to it. When discontinuing use, it's important to reduce the dosage gradually, bearing in mind that some patients may be more vulnerable to addiction than others.

MUSCLE RELAXANTS

Pain can often be accompanied by muscle spasms and cramps, especially in the case of neck and back problems following a trauma. Muscle relaxants can help to relieve painful tension and expedite healing by facilitating circulation to the injured area. However, as many relaxants—particularly cyclobenzaprine (Flexeril)—have the unfortunate effect of causing drowsiness, dizziness, and confusion, they are only available on prescription. One muscle relaxant typically available over the counter is methocarbamol (Robaxin, Robaxisal). As a general rule, over-the-counter drugs tend to have fewer side effects, primarily because they are less concentrated than drugs available only on prescription. However, it is important to remember that any drug can have side effects, so it is crucial to read the directions for use and information about potential interactions with other prescription drugs. If in doubt, ask your pharmacist for advice.

In cases of muscle cramps, a common reflex for many doctors is to prescribe muscle relaxants from the get-go. However, if the pain persists, this typically means that the ligaments are to blame. Relaxants work on the muscle and will reduce cramping in this respect, but they'll have little effect on the ligaments. Anti-inflammatories will act more effectively on inflammation and swelling. If the issue is recurrent, though, it will take more than anti-inflammatories and muscle relaxants to resolve it.

TOPICAL TRANSDERMAL CREAMS

Here's a subject that's topical in more ways than one. Relatively recently, the pharmaceutical industry has developed an array of medicated transdermal pain-relief creams and patches that are applied topically to facilitate a drug's penetration through the skin, hence the name.

It was a pharmacist by the name of Mel Alter (of the Pearson and Cohen pharmacy in Montreal) who first introduced me to these new medicated solutions around twenty years ago, at a seminar in the United States about compounds. As we saw earlier, painkillers such as morphine and its derivatives—including fentanyl—are available in the form of patches that consistently release the drug over several days. In fact, many of the other drugs described in this chapter can also be prescribed in patch or cream form for topical application. The benefits are numerous. Releasing the drug into the body in lower, consistent doses leads to fewer systemic side effects; not taking the drug orally gives the liver a break; and finally, applying cream or patches reduces the risk of overdose for patients who suffer from confusion or tend to forget to take their pills. What's more, this approach is preferable for localized pain, since the drug is concentrated in the affected area.

Manipulation techniques

Doctors don't learn about manipulating the spine and joints at medical school, yet these techniques can often be highly effective and bring about immediate results. Some mobilization is taught in orthopedics and physiotherapy, but these techniques tend not to be used frequently. Increasingly however, the various types of manipulation used in chiropractic and osteopathy are gaining ground in the treatment of muscle and joint disorders.

I distinctly recall an incident that occurred at a talk about acupuncture in Montreal led by Dr. Anton Jayasuriya, an acupuncturist and rheumatologist originally from Sri Lanka, who had invited a guest speaker from his home country to join him. I was the first to arrive for the talk and was the only attendee in the room when the guest speaker limped in and told Dr. Jayasuriya that he was in so much pain, he wouldn't be able to give his presentation. He complained that his knee hurt so much, he couldn't extend his leg, and remarked on how strange it was that this debilitating pain had come on suddenly an hour earlier as he was walking, especially as he had never experienced it before. Seeing how much pain the speaker looked to be in as he limped up to the stage, I stepped forward to offer my assistance.

I asked him if he would let me examine his knee, and he agreed. As there was already a table on the stage for demonstrating acupuncture techniques on a supine patient, I invited him to lie down and asked him a few questions. Once I had examined him and listened to his answers, I suspected that he was suffering from a meniscus tear—in other words, a piece of cartilage in the knee had broken loose and caught in the knee joint. When this happens, it can cause intense pain and interfere with the ability to walk. I simply practiced a technique to free the cartilage from the joint, and barely two minutes later the guest speaker was able to bend his knee normally again and get up and walk without pain as if nothing had happened. He was astounded, to say the least, and I received a wonderful thank-you letter from him when he got back home to Sri Lanka.

Right from the very beginning of my practice, I realized the importance of knowing the human body inside out and developing a sense of touch, manipulation, and mobilization. It's amazing what medical miracles we can accomplish with our hands—and zero medication. I have used the manual techniques I learned from Dr. James Cyriax and American osteopaths to help many patients who were suffering from neck, shoulder, ankle, or back pain, not only in my office, but also in the emergency room.

CHIROPRACTIC

Chiropractors use manual techniques to treat, diagnose, and prevent disorders of the musculoskeletal system, primarily in the spine and upper and lower limbs.

This treatment method was established over a hundred years ago by Daniel David "D. D." Palmer in Iowa. Palmer's approach was so radical at the time that he was jailed for practicing medicine without a license. Still, his practice gained recognition as early as 1897, and it was all thanks to a janitor in his office building whose hearing was impaired. Two years earlier, the janitor, Harvey Lillard, had explained to Palmer how his hearing loss had started when he made one wrong move and felt a crack in his spine. Palmer pushed the vertebra back into place, and Lillard claimed he could hear perfectly again by the very next day. Palmer, who already had an interest in non-traditional treatments, concluded that the nervous system was the key to health and determined that proper alignment of the spine was an essential part of keeping the nerve impulses flowing.

Today, chiropractic is widely recognized and legislated as a health profession in many countries, and there are chiropractic schools across North America and around the world. Chiropractors can practice legally in most European countries, where they are recognized as independent health professionals governed by various national associations under the umbrella of the European Chiropractors' Union (ECU). This practice is particularly widespread in northern mainland Europe, the United Kingdom, and the Scandinavian countries.

Chiropractic primarily addresses mechanical issues of the neuro-musculoskeletal system by treating functional disruptions referred to as **subluxations**. These slight misalignments of the vertebrae are regarded in chiropractic theory as the cause of many health problems. Chiropractors use hands-on techniques to restore balance through spinal and muscular adjustments that involve applying specific impulses to pressure points in a particular part of an osteoarticular segment, i.e., the bone and the joint. Though specific adjustments may vary depending on the chiropractic school and techniques used, several treatments are generally administered with the goal of restoring healthy function to a joint or connected organ.

Chiropractic adjustments often provide rapid, effective relief. In addition to manual adjustments, chiropractic doctors may use various complementary techniques, such as electrotherapy, massage, ultrasound, and therapy to release painful trigger points (muscle knots), as well as advising patients on healthy life choices.

However, a word of caution is in order about chiropractic adjustments that involve neck manipulation with forced extension and rotation movements. This type of manipulation may cause or aggravate pain for elderly patients with severe osteoarthritis and potentially lead to severe neurological complications due to compression or even dissection of the arteries at the base of the neck. Fortunately, these techniques are increasingly falling out of favor.

OSTEOPATHY

Osteopathy is another hands-on approach that deserves wider recognition. Though it's often described as "unconventional," this branch of alternative medicine is a profession in itself that employs manual techniques to provide perfectly safe and effective treatment for any muscle, joint, or nerve disorder. Osteopathy is often used as a complement to physiotherapy, though it doesn't use rehabilitation and strength-building programs and exercises, technology, or equipment as such.

Founded by American physician Andrew Taylor Still in 1874, the practice of osteopathy hinges on the use of manual techniques to restore mobility to the various structures of the body, recondition physiological function in the organs, and restore what we call **homeostasis**—the balance that's so important to our health. The founding principle of osteopathy is that structure governs function, and vice versa.

According to this principle, restoring the structure of an organ will enable it to regain its function. The scope of this practice therefore goes beyond simply mobilizing a muscle or joint and acknowledges the holistic nature and interconnection of the human body.

Osteopathy remains a relatively uncommon practice in Canada, although it's quite widely recognized and practiced by physicians in Europe as well as in in the United States, where doctors of osteopathy use spine and joint manipulation techniques incorporating rapid, low-amplitude movements to reposition various joints. As with many chiropractic adjustments, these movements are often accompanied by little cracking sounds that seem to indicate the adjustment has been made. However, osteopathic adjustments to the muscles, joints, and organs are very gentle—so much so that patients sometimes feel like nothing has happened, though the benefits soon become apparent. In fact, I regularly refer patients of mine to physiotherapists with osteopathy training, as the very gentle osteopathic manipulations can easily provide relief for various joint, muscle, and nerve issues.

The legal status of osteopathy varies tremendously from one country to another. In the United States, particularly the western part of the country, doctors of osteopathy (DOs) train for seven to ten years, just like medical doctors (MDs). They work in hospitals and can prescribe medicines and do general or specialized surgery. Defenders of traditional Western medicine have been hostile to osteopathic methods over the years and attempted to have osteopathy schools shut down, but these attempts failed, and the osteopathic approach lives on today.

Among the subtler techniques to stem from the meticulous, precise touch of osteopathy is craniosacral therapy. This very gentle manual technique was developed by an American osteopath, John Upledger, DO, in the 1970s. Practitioners work with the bones of the skull, vertebrae, and sacrum, applying only a very slight pressure to the patient's body. This allows them to sense the wavelike movement of energy—craniosacral rhythms—in the body, and gently palpate the affected bones and limbs to re-establish the flow where energy is stuck. Craniosacral therapy is suitable for patients of all ages, from young babies to the elderly, and there are no contraindications.

The subtlety of this technique belies its power to free patients of pain, physical tension, and even psychological stress. You really have to try it to see how effective such a gentle approach can be. I have attended a number of training courses on this form of therapy in the United States and Europe, and I can attest that even though medical and scientific evidence may be lacking, it has brought relief and even accelerated the healing process for many of my patients, who are often surprised at how I can examine and treat them using the very gentlest of movements.

MASSAGE

We humans have always used our hands to apply pressure to our bodies and rub pain away. Just like animals instinctively lick their wounds, we are programmed to touch and feel wherever our body hurts. Over the ages, various techniques have emerged, developed, and grown in popularity. Today's therapeutic massage techniques can help to improve our quality of life in many ways: providing a sense of relaxation; treating sports injuries; reducing swelling in limbs following surgery; relieving muscle pain, tension, and spasms; soothing injured and torn ligaments; alleviating arthritis symptoms; restoring movement; and relieving headaches and migraines.

Massage involves applying pressure with movement, primarily to skin, muscle, and ligament tissue. The health benefits and physiological effects are plentiful. Massage can stimulate blood flow and increase joint mobility, reduce blood pressure, and promote physical and mental relaxation.

Generally speaking, massage has an effect on the parasympathetic nervous system by allowing it to rest and relax. It also calms the sympathetic nervous system and alleviates the symptoms of restlessness associated with fear and danger. Massage can relieve pain and reduce levels of the stress hormone cortisol. It offers significant benefits for sleep quality and well-being by stimulating the "happy" neurotransmitters we call endorphins, dopamine, and serotonin. However, I cannot extol the virtues of massage without stressing the importance of an informed, attentive, and compassionate therapist.

Today, the science of massage is increasingly widely recognized, and there are plenty of options in countries around the world for anyone to learn the basics and see the benefits. Massage is the science of touch, and we humans are very receptive to the touch of a well-meaning loved one. By this token, mothers who massage their babies will surely see the benefits in their physical, mental, and psychological development.

One of the greatest benefits of massage is the sense of relaxation and well-being it can bring for the mind as well as the body. When I give massage therapy treatments to relieve pain, it's not uncommon for patients to cry. Touching certain muscle areas that are tense can bring painful experiences flooding back, and the tears come flowing as the psychological suffering that has accumulated in these muscles is released.

Some believe the body is a giant field of feelings, where every part of the body harbors a particular emotion. Several books have even published entire lists of illnesses and ailments thought to be rooted in hidden emotions. I've been fortunate to meet practitioners who claimed they could "decode," so to speak, any physical symptom and connect it to a particular emotion. The challenge lies in pinpointing the precise meaning of an emotional connection, however, since not all psychological causes can possibly be taken at face value with respect to a diseased organ. It's important not to generalize, however; there is no single cause for any ailment that applies for everyone, which is why every treatment must be personalized. However, when there is a legitimate relationship, helping patients to pinpoint the root cause of their ailment—which may often be emotional—can be enormously beneficial. After all, we are both body and mind, and our muscles and organs have the capacity to act like sponges, absorbing the psychological tension we feel.

Let's explore the benefits of using therapeutic massage to treat pain.

Deep massage and trigger points (muscle knots)

A gentle, relaxing massage can certainly help to relieve stress and muscle cramps. However, massage therapy really comes into its own when we go deep into the muscles, and there's nothing like deep pressure-point massage when it comes to getting rid of chronic muscle pain and muscle knots. Knots are fibrous bands in the muscle, generally easy to find by simply palpating the area. Some of these contractures are extremely sensitive to deep palpation and can trigger remote pain.

The late Dr. Janet Travell (1901–1997) was an American researcher who delved deep into the issue of muscle disorders and pain manifestation.[3] I had the pleasure of meeting her at a symposium when she was eighty years old. Dr. Travell demonstrated how certain parts of a muscle, when injured, can produce remote pain, referred to as **myofascial pain syndrome** (MPS). ("Myofascial" has nothing to do with the face—fascia are the envelopes that surround the muscles and other organs, and the "myo" prefix refers to something related to a muscle.)

MPS may occur following trauma or overuse of certain muscles. Dr. Travell's work alludes to the role of trigger points as the source of this referred pain and demonstrates how treating these trigger points through the use of manipulation, massage, or injections can eliminate the remote pain. These impressive achievements earned Dr. Travell the honor of becoming the personal physician of President John F. Kennedy, who suffered from intense back pain following injuries he sustained in the Second World War.

One frequently encountered example of myofascial pain syndrome is a real pain in the butt—a knot (painful induration) in the gluteal muscle that causes pain in the thigh or elsewhere in the leg. Typically a cursory assessment of the knee or thigh reveals nothing, but in a broader examination intense pain is discovered in the buttock. When that muscle is massaged and pressure is applied, the pain spreads down into the leg and knee. It's as if the muscle fibers had contracted in a part of the muscle in a strange way. These stubborn knots can be undone by massaging the area, applying ice, and often administering injections to the painful muscle mass. Dr. Travell developed and often combined a number of simple, painless injection and massage techniques to treat these trigger points.

Paul was a patient of mine who consulted for pain in his lumbar spine and left thigh that had persisted for months. He had tried massage treatments for his entire lower back and thigh and had also taken anti-inflammatories, but nothing had really worked. When I examined him, I found some knots in the gluteal muscle, and when I palpated these deeply he writhed and twisted in pain. Paul told me that the pressure I had applied to the muscle knot had triggered an intense pain in his thigh, right where he had been experiencing the chronic pain. I massaged the area deeply—which was a little uncomfortable for us both at times—and slowly released the knot in the gluteal muscle. Gradually Paul felt the blood flow to his thigh increase, and the pain disappeared. After two further massage treatments, even the lumbar pain disappeared, since it was likely the product of overcompensation by the gluteal muscles. This kind of chronic lumbar and leg pain can often ensue following muscle tension in the pelvic area.

How trigger points relate to leg and buttock pain

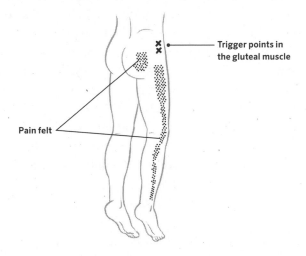

Trigger points in
the gluteal muscle

Pain felt

This illustration shows the pain path from the buttock to the thigh and lower leg. This pain stems from the trigger points marked xx above the area where the pain is felt, which the patient may often not automatically describe as painful. However, when deep pressure is applied to the muscle in the xx area, the patient may describe feeling a pain down the entire leg.

A short word of caution about fibromyalgia: While massages are generally harmless, certain precautions should still be taken. A deep massage may trigger muscle pain for certain patients, and worse still, that pain may persist for several days following the massage. Based on my experience, one group of patients likely to be poor candidates for deep massage are fibromyalgia sufferers. Not only is their capacity to eliminate toxins and lactic acid likely to be significantly diminished, but also the pressure on the muscle may tend to be a source of pain during the massage itself. This technique is thus best avoided in such circumstances, unless the massage is very short and gentle.

Another word of caution for patients on blood thinners: Too vigorous a massage may lead to local hemorrhaging and even severe hematoma. Patients taking the blood thinner warfarin (Coumadin) are particularly at risk, since this drug increases bleeding time, and a muscle that is oozing even slightly may cause excessive bleeding. Individuals taking a low-dose aspirin (81 mg) will not typically be vulnerable to increased bleeding. However, they would be wise to avoid some overly keen and energetic massage therapists, since even without the effect of heavy-duty blood thinners, they may experience some nasty bruising.

An important word of caution about infections and cancer: Massaging an infected area of the body is strictly contraindicated. There is a risk that the massage will spread the infection deeper and lead to more severe inflammation. The same goes for cancer patients. These individuals can still enjoy a massage, but must avoid any massaging of the area where the cancer is located as well as areas that may be affected by metastasis. The following techniques may be better suited to these conditions, which warrant a more cautious approach.

Scar massage

After surgery, scars can take a long time to disappear, as the tissue can tend to thicken, harden, and retract. It can be helpful to go for massages—or to practice self-massage techniques, if the scar is easy to reach—to soften the scar tissue on the surface as well as at a deeper level. Using almond oil or vitamin E oil during the massage can promote elasticity and vascularization of the surrounding tissue. Because scars can also cause referred pain, it's important to treat them properly. If no curative effects are observed, injections at the scar site may be required.

Deep transverse friction massage (DTFM)

This underused massage technique can bring about surprising results, and the good news is, you can do it yourself. Following an established diagnosis of tendinitis or ligamentitis, deep transverse friction massage can provide relief and often promote complete healing. If the ligament has suffered microtearing, it can be prevented from healing properly. DTFM works by triggering a temporary inflammatory response, which stimulates circulation and frees the microadhesions to allow the ligament to heal.

It's easy to do, and it's highly effective. Using your thumb or index finger, gently massage the whole length of the ligament using a transverse motion. After a few minutes, you can increase the pressure, but not so much that it feels too uncomfortable. Generally, seven to eight minutes at a time will suffice, because it's important to avoid creating too severe a reaction. To ensure sufficient time to recover, this treatment should be repeated every other day for two to three weeks. *You can see a demonstration of this technique on my website at drbrouillard.com.*

Knee massage

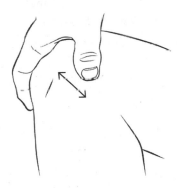

Elbow massage

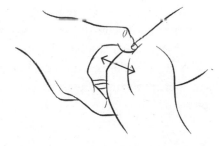

Ice massage

Here's another basic technique that can provide rapid relief and even promote healing. However, this approach does require a certain degree of muscle knowledge, which is easy enough to acquire by looking at the shape and position of the muscles on an anatomical chart. Generally speaking, the muscles follow the form of the long bones. In other words, the forearm muscles go from the elbow to the wrist, and the leg muscles go from the pelvis to the knee and from the knee to the foot. All you need is an ice cube to soothe that painful muscle, though you may find it more comfortable to fill a Styrofoam cup with water and freeze it to make an ice pack instead.

Engage the muscle and stretch it to the maximum, then use a slow sliding motion along the length of the muscle fibers to apply pressure. Stretching and massaging the muscle under this sliding pressure, along with the effect of the cold, will ultimately help to relax it and heal the painful tension. This technique can be used for about ten minutes and should be repeated twice a day for two weeks. Personally, like many physiotherapy schools, I use a "stretch and spray" technique, which involves first stretching the muscle and then slowly spraying a very cold solution along the length of the muscle fibers.

Injections

Over the course of my career, I've administered more than 100,000 injections to relieve pain, to my patients' great benefit. In the capable hands of a physician, rheumatologist, orthopedist, or anesthesiologist, these techniques can rapidly deliver impressive results. For treatment to be effective, it's important to clarify the diagnosis, determine the cause, and pinpoint the precise location of the injury. This technique is facilitated today by the use of ultrasound to guide the needle. Let's take a quick look at some of the injection techniques and substances used to treat chronic pain.

LOCAL AND REGIONAL INJECTIONS

This technique involves injecting the treatment product directly into a joint, tendon, ligament, or muscle knot. For spinal pain issues caused by osteoarthritis, injections known as joint blocks may be administered to the facet joints, which are the joints between the vertebrae.

In cases of a herniated disc, epidural injections may be administered to treat the area around the compressed nerve root. This approach works on the same principle as an epidural used during childbirth. A **foraminal epidural** is an injection to the exit of a spinal nerve and a **caudal epidural** is an injection to the end of the sacrum. As a general rule, the use of an anesthetic may release local compression, whereas the use of cortisone will reduce inflammatory phenomena, easing sciatic pain in the case of injections to the lumbar area.

Some pain may be attributed to abnormal activity in the sympathetic nervous system, which, as part of its role in defending the body, may bombard an injured area. For example, an arm fracture may cause pain all the way down the arm to the hand, and reduced circulation may cause symptoms of cold and discoloration. A series of sympathetic nerve blocks (injections of an anesthetic) can settle the nerve and bring it back to normal. I once treated a nurse who had developed this regional syndrome as a reaction to a jab in her arm for a vaccination. After two months of injections and acupuncture treatments, everything settled back to normal.

TRIGGER POINT (MUSCLE KNOT) INJECTIONS

Discovering Dr. Janet Travell's research and breakthroughs on trigger points (page 131) was a major revelation for me. Injecting xylocaine directly into a muscle trigger point, which allows the muscle to release completely, will make the pain disappear immediately. With preventive exercise, it often will not return. To restore greater muscle function, anti-inflammatory ingredients and collagen may be added.

I can recall some patients who felt no pain at all in the muscle that was the actual source of their injury. They complained of pain elsewhere in the body without realizing the muscle that was to blame was painful as well. I remember one patient in particular who was convinced she was suffering a migraine headache, though that turned out not to be the case. When I examined and pinched her sternocleidomastoid muscle—a muscle in the neck that allows us to turn our head—she experienced a sharp pain, and I could feel a hardened area, a little like a piece of rope. I administered an injection to the muscle, where, through palpation, I had felt the most hardness—this is usually in the larger, red part of the muscle—and the headache disappeared completely.

Muscle tension is one of the most frequent causes of headaches and neck or back pain—a problem many people suffer from these days, as our fast pace of life and lack of rest, relaxation, and exercise make us easy prey.

CORTISONE INJECTIONS

Many readers will already be familiar with the anti-inflammatory cortisone. Cortisone injections are often sufficient to relieve acute pain caused by conditions such as bursitis of the shoulder, for example. However, when the pain persists and becomes chronic, I've observed that a different approach is often necessary, because cortisone can have undesirable effects in the long term. Other treatments may be considered when cortisone is no longer working or when it's contraindicated.

CORTISONE

Cortisone is a word that still fills many of us with fear, yet it provides pain relief for millions of people every day. Cortisone is a natural part of our molecular makeup. Produced by the adrenal glands, it's a precursor to cortisol, the so-called "stress hormone" we seem to be hearing about more and more. Cortisone has been used in medicine for at least the last seventy-five years, and it's an ingredient in almost every drug cocktail.

Cortisone sometimes gets a bad rap because it's used too often, at too high a dose, or for too long a time. Indeed, its risks can be numerous, including osteoporosis, damaged tendon fibers, reduced immune resistance, weight gain, heightened diabetes, glandular imbalance, heart disease, hypertension, and depression, to name but a few.

These are the same symptoms patients can suffer when tumors stimulate the adrenal glands. When we're stressed, we produce cortisol, which can be just as destructive as cortisone, with all the same side effects we want to avoid. Many of us don't realize just how destructive stress can be; like chronic inflammation, it's a silent killer. It's become almost an obsession for me to warn people about the psychological and physical damage stress can cause.

Cortisone, however, is an important drug. It's invaluable in the event of anaphylactic shock for individuals with severe allergies as well as being an excellent anti inflammatory and antiallergic drug. Used occasionally in low doses—no more than three times per year—in a given area it can be highly beneficial and is not dangerous. As with any other drug, it's important to heed the indications and dosage and frequency instructions.

Cortisone is often the preferred treatment for persistent acute inflammation before moving on to different injectable solutions. It can be administered by injection or in oral tablet form, depending on the circumstances. In any case, it remains important not only to treat the side effects of the inflammation but also to identify the source of the inflammation and treat its cause.

HYALURONIC ACID INJECTIONS (VISCOSUPPLEMENTATION)

Hyaluronic acid injections were first used in the 1970s to help restore lost vitreous humor—the clear, jellylike substance in the eye—following eye surgery. Their use was then extended to treat osteoarthritis, primarily of the knee, followed some years later by the ankles and hips. Some twenty years ago, I was able to observe its benefits for shoulder issues too.

This treatment involves injecting an elastic, viscous substance containing hyaluronic acid—such as Synvisc, Durolane, Hyalgan, or Suplasyn—into the joint. As well as being the primary component of synovial fluid (a superb natural lubricant that protects the cartilage and contributes to tissue hydration and cohesion), hyaluronic acid bears similarities to collagen, though it is more concentrated in cartilage, tendons, and joints. Injecting hyaluronic acid boosts joint viscosity and elasticity while helping to reduce the degeneration of cartilage as well as inflammation in the joint. This makes it a useful technique for reducing osteoarthritis pain.

Hyaluronic acid has grown quickly in popularity as a facial anti-wrinkle treatment by acting as a filler. Whether we use them to relieve joint pain or to smooth our skin, hyaluronic acid injections can only be a temporary solution and will need to be repeated in the months and years that follow.

PROLOTHERAPY

In the introduction to this book, I mentioned what a key role my encounter with the late Dr. James Cyriax in the 1980s had played in shaping my education as a physician specializing in musculoskeletal issues. Besides standard cortisone injections, Dr. Cyriax used an injection-based treatment known as prolotherapy (short for proliferation therapy). Although numerous physicians and pain-treatment clinics successfully practice this technique across the United States and Canada, it's yet to gain widespread use and recognition.

Prolotherapy is a simple and effective technique that involves injecting a substance containing dextrose (sugar) and xylocaine (a mild analgesic) into the painful attachment points of tendons or ligaments. One of the advantages of using xylocaine is that the way it works makes the injection itself pain free. What's more, it can easily confirm that the exact source of the problem has been pinpointed because right after treatment, patients often marvel that their pain has gone away.

The concentration of glucose used in prolotherapy is typically 12 to 15 percent, which is two to three times the normal level in the human body (5 percent). While it isn't enough to raise our blood sugar, this increased concentration of glucose triggers a mild, acute, and transitory inflammatory reaction at the injection site. This reaction sets a chain of biochemical repair and regeneration processes in motion—hence the term "proliferation"—to promote deep healing of the injured tendons and ligaments.

By enabling the tissues to regenerate, prolotherapy helps to relieve the pain from chronic sprains and tendinitis and has proven to be an effective treatment for osteoarthritis, back pain, tendinitis, bursitis, partial tendon tears, epicondylitis (tennis elbow), sciatica, and many other conditions.[4] It's particularly effective in treating painful stretched ligaments. Frequently, individuals who have suffered a succession of sprains may experience a chronic disruption of ligament structure. Sprained ankles are a common example: after several injuries, the swelling tends to persist in the ankle, which leads to pain when walking. Physical rehabilitation does nothing to ease the pain, and surgery is of little use either. Fortunately, however, these types of partial ligament injuries—often with microcracks—tend to respond favorably to prolotherapy treatment.

During my travels in Europe and the United States, I've found prolotherapy to be widely used, especially when treating elite athletes. Here in Canada, some of my colleagues in sports medicine have come to me to pick my brain about this technique, and I've told them how effective it can be, even in complex and chronic scenarios, and what a safe treatment it is. Even repeated injections have no undesirable side effects, unlike with steroid compounds such as cortisone.

Prolotherapy has proven to be an effective treatment in this kind of scenario even for professional dancers and Olympic champions who were referred to me for persistent pain and physical incapacity.

Taking prolotherapy to the next level

Over the years and depending on local availability, various substances have been added to the standard dextrose-xylocaine mix to enhance its effectiveness, including collagen, interleukins, fibrin, endorphins, and growth factors. These elements stimulate microcirculation as well as the production of new collagen fibers supporting the connective tissue. Persistent lower back pain following an operation on the lumbar discs tends to respond well to these techniques.

Platelet-rich plasma (PRP) injections, which use the patient's own plasma, are another similar, albeit expensive, treatment growing in popularity with sports medicine practitioners and beauty therapists.[5] Blood platelets contain bioactive protein and growth factors. This technique involves collecting a small quantity of the patient's blood and spinning it in a centrifuge. As the red blood cells fall to the bottom of the tube, the clear plasma, which is very high in fibrins and growth factors, rises to the top and can be extracted. Autologous—meaning the patient's own—plasma is used in beauty therapy for various purposes, from promoting hair regrowth to improving facial skin texture. From a medical perspective, autologous plasma can be injected into a ligament in the same way as glucose and dextrose and is regarded as a proliferation therapy technique, although the centrifugation process makes it much more expensive. What's more, these substances can be injected closer to the surface, at cutaneous level into acupuncture points. This simple technique is called **biopuncture**. As for acupuncture, we'll explore that a little later in this chapter.

Dr. Cyriax deconstructed the way joints work, which made it possible to determine, in the case of a shoulder condition, for instance, whether the problem stemmed from a muscle, tendon, ligament, or capsule. It was fascinating to see how being able to pinpoint the exact source of the pain and treat it with injections instead of a trial-and-error approach led to such amazing results; the more precisely the injections were targeted, the more effective the healing process became.

Back then, in the early 1980s, ultrasound was not as widely used as it is today, so any manipulations and injections required a very advanced level of anatomical knowledge. Today, ultrasound is used to check the condition of soft tissue (tendons, muscles, and sometimes ligaments), but it alone cannot form the basis for treatment. Instead, the patient must present clinical signs and symptoms that point to the source of the injury, and the ultrasound then serves to confirm the diagnosis. Another advantage of ultrasound is that it enables the needle to be guided precisely to the target anatomical site in the case of complex injection techniques or patient obesity.

ONE PAINLESS TECHNIQUE

I myself am sensitive to pain, and this has led me to develop needle-puncture injection techniques that cause very little pain (and often none at all). I figure my sensitivity stems from a number of childhood experiences with dentists who caused me to suffer a terrible amount of pain. One episode in particular has always been engraved in my mind.

When I was ten years old, my mother took me to the dentist for pain in one of my upper left molars. The dentist examined me, and as soon as he had located the cavity, he decided to extract the tooth. Back then, dentists—at least those who were unsure of themselves—tended to pull teeth out rather than repair them. It was my first such experience, and as I was still young and naive, I nodded to confirm I understood what was happening. After the dentist told me he was going to yank out my tooth, I figured the tooth was hurting anyway so I had nothing to lose. The dentist was a man of few words and seemed to be somewhat nervous and a little hurried.

I remember feeling the pain of the needle piercing my gum, followed by an unpleasant pressure right by my painful tooth. Since I was a brave young man, I simply grimaced and forced a smile. A few minutes later, which seemed to be nowhere near long enough to me, he returned, probably with pliers in his hand. I didn't dare look, in any case. He told me to open my mouth wide—no, wider, he said. Then I felt the pliers take hold around my somewhat desensitized tooth. The dentist pulled down on the tooth, but it resisted stubbornly and I could feel the pain growing. The more the tooth held on, the more intense the pain became as the dentist pushed and pulled at it. I started to wonder who would win this tug-of-war!

The pain was becoming unbearable, and apparently I was starting to pale somewhat. "Don't tell me he's going to pass out," the dentist quipped to my mother. As I sweated buckets in the torture chair, he suddenly grabbed my head and shoved it down between my legs. "That'll help with your blood pressure so you don't faint," he said to me. I didn't know it at the time, but that was the first thing I learned about medicine. Lesson number one: pain can make a patient lose consciousness. Lesson number two: positioning the head below the heart promotes blood flow to the brain. Lesson number three: better circulation to the brain avoids loss of consciousness. Because that's precisely what happened: I didn't pass out (unfortunately for me). When the moment had passed, the dentist lifted my head back up and asked me to open my mouth again, even wider. I could feel the metal jaws of the pliers clamped firmly around my tooth. The dentist yanked down on the tooth, but still it resisted. I was really starting to panic at this point, because the pain was excruciating and the whole left side of my head was hurting. I could smell the dentist's breath as he leaned in closer and braced his leg against the chair to get more leverage. I braced myself and suffered like a martyr before finally breathing a sigh of relief as all was calm once more. The dentist stood up and looked in astonishment at his pliers, then told my mother and me that he had ended up pulling out two teeth for the price of one! The roots were apparently entangled, so one wouldn't come out without the other.

Following this excruciatingly painful experience, a good ten years went by before I dared to visit a dentist again—obviously not the same one as before. For a long time, I was afraid of needles. Fortunately, though, a cousin of mine is a dentist and his gentle approach to treatment helped to appease my fears. I have since gone on to work with a great dentist in Montreal, Dr. Daniel Laramée, who uses a holistic biocompatible and functional approach to dentistry.

That childhood experience in the dentist's chair left lasting scars in my mind. Observing surgical procedures in my third year of medical school would often make me feel queasy, so I had to reprogram the way I saw flesh, blood, and needles. With time, I went on to be able to carry out surgical procedures ably, confidently, and effectively and deal with the worst possible kinds of trauma in the emergency room.

The upside of my misadventure at the dentist's office is that I've always taken extreme precautions to avoid my own patients feeling pain. Often, patients tell me they felt nothing at all when I gave them an injection. I typically use topical aerosol and intradermal anesthetics, and before ultrafine needles were available in Canada, I used to order them from Europe and the United States. Using very fine needles can prevent vasovagal shock—fainting of the patient—which isn't a pleasant experience for the patient or the doctor. I've always taken the time it takes to insert a needle, to the point where I've been able to feel when the needle was ready to go deeper without causing the patient any pain. I've even suggested to some very fearful patients that they try to visualize the needle entering the skin very gently.

Patients with fibromyalgia may experience an unpleasant feeling with muscle injections, not due to the needle being inserted, but because the injected substance creates pressure in the muscle. In fact, this reaction can be an indicator that a patient may have fibromyalgia, even in the absence of other factors. With all fibromyalgia sufferers, it's important to inject the substance very slowly to ensure the patient feels no unduly unpleasant pressure, even if the pain for which they consulted will have almost completely disappeared a few minutes later.

Acupuncture

Acupuncture is another form of treatment that uses needles, but in a very different way, as it doesn't involve injections, and the fine needles used in acupuncture have a gentler, blunt tip. Acupuncture can be an effective treatment for a great many ailments, including spinal, joint, and muscle conditions, neck pain, headaches, and lingering pain following a sprained ankle, as well as menstrual disorders and allergies. And in contrast to a drug-based approach, acupuncture is a form of bio-energetic medicine that treats the whole person and aims to restore balance in the body.

Because I'm curious by nature, I've always enjoyed researching and exploring various treatment options, many of which have been highly effective with no side effects. I started my acupuncture studies in 1981, and pain relief was what initially drew me to the field. The more I studied acupuncture, the more I realized it offered solutions to all kinds of problems.

The most obvious potential stumbling block for acupuncture is fear of the needle, or the sensation of the needle itself, which some patients may find unpleasant. Generally, however, acupuncture is a pain-free treatment.

IS ACUPUNCTURE
A MEDICAL PRACTICE?

Acupuncture is now widely recognized by medical authorities, and many private insurance plans cover acupuncture treatments. In Canada and the United States, the practice of acupuncture is regulated in many provinces and states by various professional associations and governing bodies. In Europe, regulations vary and many countries have professional associations for acupuncturists.

Josie was a patient I saw for an urgent appointment around eight-thirty one evening. A mother of two who had otherwise always been in good health, she had gone to the emergency room that afternoon complaining of a headache so intense that her usual treatment of acetaminophen and ibuprofen could not shift it. Josie told me that the ER doctor had examined her carefully, told her that she was suffering a migraine attack, given her an injection of Demerol (a morphine-like painkiller) that had only provided temporary relief, and sent her home with a prescription.

She decided to consult with me and try alternative treatment, because the pain on the left side of her head was still excruciating and made her feel nauseous and very sensitive to light. She walked into my office with her eyes half-closed and her husband guiding her forward. I suggested that we start with an osteopathic treatment to remodel the cranial and cervical area, and after barely fifteen minutes, to even my great surprise, Josie experienced a wave of relief. I then inserted a few acupuncture needles, and the pain and various symptoms went away completely and never came back. This may seem like a miracle cure, but acupuncture and osteopathy work in an often surprising way and can bring benefits that still defy the logic of conventional medicine.

Needless to say, acupuncture is a potent weapon in my pain-treatment arsenal. I even pack acupuncture needles whenever I travel, because I never know when I might need them myself or to treat family and friends. My wife, Carole, suffers frequent migraines, and acupuncture has provided her with great relief. When she starts to see the warning signs of a migraine attack, such as blurry vision, I bring out my needles, and the symptoms can disappear after barely ten minutes, without any medication.

THE SCIENCE OF ACUPUNCTURE

Can a needle really be all it takes to relieve pain? One tiny needle, inserted in just the right place, with no injection and no drugs? You'd be forgiven for being skeptical. How can a needle eliminate pain? Is it by magic? Is there a placebo effect? Does it work by distraction? Is it really hypnosis in disguise? It can be hard to rationalize.

The mechanics of acupuncture are complex, but we can explore some of the key nuts and bolts here. Although scientific studies have been unable to explain the phenomenon, acupuncture creates an overall analgesic effect by boosting endorphins and serotonin levels. This ability of acupuncture to relieve pain in general is what first drew me to it as a treatment option, though I soon saw how its therapeutic effects went much further than simple pain relief.

Acupuncture also has a general **homeostatic** effect, meaning that it creates or restores balance in the body, mainly by acting to regulate the endocrine and nervous systems. As well as having a serotonergic effect—creating a serene and calm mood, which combats allergies, among other things—it can promote relaxation for patients with high blood pressure. Acupuncture is undeniably helpful for relieving muscle spasms and increasing circulation through the widening of blood vessels. It also regulates hormones and can treat metabolic conditions such as menstrual irregularities and mild hypothyroidism.[6]

Acupuncture is also known to play a therapeutic role in treating inflammatory conditions such as arthritis and tendinitis, since it increases cortisol levels. A temporary increase in cortisol has an anti-inflammatory effect and is surely the best natural cortisone for the body. However, a constantly high level of cortisol can be inflammatory for the whole body.

Finally, let's not forget how acupuncture benefits the immune system by stimulating the production of gamma globulins (antibodies that determine immunity), thus providing greater protection against infection.

ENERGY MERIDIANS

Acupuncture is first and foremost a regulator for the body that acts through the energy channels—meridians—that constitute a key concept of Traditional Chinese Medicine (TCM). TCM is based on a number of core philosophies, the most important being that the universe is one indivisible entity where all exists in harmony and interdependence. The body is seen as a microcosm of this vast entity that obeys the same laws. Harmony of body and mind is achieved when the two primordial forces of yin and yang—and by extension, hot and cold; light and dark; active and passive; and male and female energy—are in balance.

According to TCM, there are twelve main energy meridians in the body that connect the deep organs, and acupuncture works by stimulating specific points along these meridians. By restoring the balance between yin and yang, acupuncture helps to maintain the vital energy we need to be healthy.

We don't know exactly how the hundreds of acupuncture points were mapped out more than three thousand years ago, but we do know they exist. Electronic detectors have measured a lower skin resistance over acupuncture points, allowing them to be pinpointed even without prior knowledge of their location.[7] Somehow, the points we are able to detect with today's complex electronic instruments and those that were discovered thousands of years ago are one and the same.

NEEDLES

Acupuncturists use needles of different lengths depending on the area being treated. Often 1.2 inches is the standard needle length used, and this will typically be inserted to a depth of 0.6 inches. Some parts of the body, including the buttocks, will call for a longer needle, perhaps 2 inches in length. The most commonly used needles are made from stainless steel with a copper handle. Most acupuncturists use disposable needles, and some U.S. states have made the use of disposable needles mandatory. Hopefully this practice will become generalized, since the quality of current sterilization techniques varies too much in my opinion.

Generally, five to ten treatments will suffice to provide patients with effective, lasting relief. However, here as elsewhere, some patients will be better candidates for acupuncture than others. If no improvement is seen after six or seven sessions, treatment should be discontinued.

Because the needles are flexible, blunt-tipped, and very fine gauge, they cause very little discomfort when inserted and rarely cause bleeding when removed. Serious complications such as infections and organ punctures are very rare. Once inserted, needles are typically stimulated manually, though one technique called **electro-acupuncture** uses electrical pulses and a device similar to the TENS (transcutaneous electrical nerve stimulator) unit common in physiotherapy. Treatments usually last twenty to thirty minutes, and patients may sit upright or lie on their back. The session itself should always be restful and provide a sense of well-being. In fact, it's not uncommon for patients to fall asleep during treatment.

Children respond well to acupuncture. Because needles may be a challenge for very young children, the use of electrostimulators or lasers at the acupuncture points can be an effective and painless alternative. I have developed a completely painless technique for inserting acupuncture needles, even for young children, which involves helping the child to get used to the sensation and embrace it. As practitioners, everything hinges on our approach and the empathy we have. Our attitude can make a big difference when it comes to building the confidence of patients (and especially children) in subsequent treatments.

As you can see, acupuncture can be an attractive form of therapy with no major undesirable effects and plenty of treatment avenues to explore. We're still barely scratching the surface when it comes to understanding how this several-thousand-year-old practice works, and as new developments emerge, various pressure, color, laser, and injection techniques may add to its scope of practice.

ACUPRESSURE: ACUPUNCTURE
WITHOUT THE NEEDLES

Acupuncture points in the body can be stimulated even without the use of needles by massage and manual pressure. This simple, painless technique is known as acupressure and can be practiced by anyone. It shares similarities with shiatsu, a Japanese practice meaning "finger pressure." Here are some acupressure points we can all use to relieve certain kinds of tension, wherever we are.

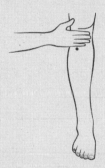

Let's start with the magic acupuncture point, **Stomach 36 (ST 36)**. Known as "Leg Three Miles" or "the point of a hundred diseases," this point can work wonders to re-energize the body and help us feel better every morning.

While it can have a beneficial effect on digestion in general, ST 36 primarily boosts vitality in all the body's organs and helps to keep us going when we're tired (hence the name). It's said to be the point of rejuvenation, prevention, and longevity. All you have to do is massage it or alternate applying and releasing pressure for five minutes. Do this every day, breathing deeply into and out of your belly. You'll see the changes happen gradually. Below are some other points that can be just as beneficial.

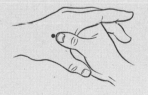

For pain in general, headaches, migraines, and dental pain, the point is **Large Intestine 4 (LI 4)**.

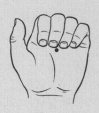

For chest pain, tightness, and anxiety, the point is **Pericardium 8 (P8)**.

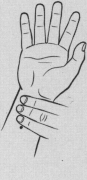

For pregnancy-related nausea and motion sickness, the point is **Pericardium 6 (P6)**.

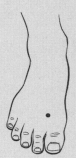

For back pain and arterial hypertension, the **Liver 3 (LV 3)** point on the top of the foot can also be very effective.

Magnetic field therapy

Late one Saturday night, around a quarter to midnight, snow was falling gently outside as I sat comfortably in the living room watching the end of a movie—and then the phone rang.

It was late, but I picked it up anyway. "Hello..."

"Hi, Gaétan."

"Oh, hi, Pierre, what's up?" I wondered why my friend was calling at this hour.

"I'm at the hospital. I had a bad fall skiing this afternoon up at Mont-Tremblant. It was pretty serious, so they took me to the ER. The doctor diagnosed a serious hip fracture and referred me to the Maisonneuve-Rosemont Hospital in Montreal for an operation."

"Well, I can see they're taking care of you," I replied, keen to get back to my movie. "You know I work there too, and they have some of the best orthopedic hip surgeons, so you're in good hands."

"Yes, well, that's the problem," Pierre replied. "The surgeon wants to give me a complete hip replacement. I'm only forty-nine, and those replacements barely last fifteen to twenty years, especially for someone as active as me. I'd have to get another hip replacement done in fifteen years and that would be much more complicated. I know you have one of those pulsed electromagnetic field machines that can help to rebuild bone and cartilage, and you've told me what a great therapy it is. I really don't want a complete hip replacement. Can you please help me find another solution?"

"Let me see. I'd like to talk to the orthopedist first," I said.

The orthopedist told me Pierre had suffered a fracture to the upper femoral area of the hip, where the bone is thin, and confirmed that he was planning to do a complete hip replacement.

"If the femoral head is intact, why not try to pin it with a plate and screws?" I asked.

"A simpler operation with screws won't hold up in that area," the surgeon explained. "The bone is too thin and fragile, and I know from experience that it won't fuse properly and might not heal fully. Especially because he's so active, a repair like that would only last three to six months before it needed fixing again."

I relayed all this to Pierre, but he was adamant he wanted to avoid major surgery. After he and I talked to his surgeon, Pierre decided to go with the plate-and-screw pinning operation; he signed a treatment waiver declining the hip replacement and absolving the surgeon from his medical duty. I would then follow up with pulsed electromagnetic field (PEMF) treatments as soon as he was able to come in to my office.

And so, after three weeks of keeping weight off his legs, Pierre limped his way into my office on crutches. We started the PEMF therapy and continued five days a week for a total of twelve treatments. Pierre felt great and was no longer in any pain. He went for an initial follow-up X-ray and, to the surgeon's great surprise, the fracture had healed. The surgeon even showed the results to a colleague to boast about the success of his plate-and-screw surgery and how well it had healed, beyond all medical expectations.

When Pierre went back for a second follow-up, another X-ray confirmed that everything had healed properly and was perfectly solid, and the surgeon told Pierre he could start his normal activities again. Much to the surgeon's astonishment, Pierre admitted that he had been pedaling up a storm on his bike for a while already and had even gone for hikes up the mountain. That was more than twelve years ago, and now Pierre is still as active as always and continues to enjoy skiing and other sports without any restriction of movement.

I've used the same magnetic field therapy that helped Pierre to help numerous other patients, sometimes even elderly patients who were suffering from osteoarthritis and experienced a remarkable degree of pain relief.[8] It's a simple technique. The patient sits comfortably or relaxes in a reclined position. The area to be treated is placed for an hour inside a cylinder that generates magnetic fields. These fields stimulate the cells, which are electrically polarized. This gives the cells a very gentle workout, which brings about increased vascularization and decreased inflammation, and promotes healing.

In general, about a dozen of these treatments will suffice. Patients who have undergone a hip replacement that fails to heal properly even after six months—who would normally have to try a second bone graft—can experience lasting bone healing after just a few weeks of treatment. This safe, painless technique has been used to relieve many kinds of chronic inflammatory pain. It has long been recognized in Europe, where it's used by more than three hundred physiotherapy clinics and doctors—I first heard about this device and its benefits at least twenty years ago from a group of German doctors. I've used PEMF therapy to obtain some very encouraging results for osteoarthritis in elderly patients. The magnetic field technique is especially renowned for treating animals—and notably racehorses' knees. The device is approved by the Therapeutic Products Directorate of Health Canada and as time goes on, we're sure to find out more about why it works.

Pulsed electromagnetic fields were first discovered in the early 1900s by none other than Nikola Tesla. Today's medical world could have benefited tremendously from this great modern inventor's discoveries in terms of joint pathology and many other health conditions. Tesla invented various magnetic field techniques for treating a range of conditions with no side effects. But the American government strong-armed these inventions, and they have long since been forgotten. Today, we're all familiar with Tesla electric cars and ultra-fast charging stations for electric vehicles. Perhaps one day charging stations like these will exist for humans to keep us in good health without resorting to medication.

Reflexology

A few years ago, my wife and I were traveling in Thailand, the Land of Smiles, and were making our way to the northern city of Chiang Mai. It was getting late, and we managed to jump on the last train of the day, which would take six hours to get us to our destination. We were surprised to see that we were some of the only passengers aboard the old train. Sitting across from one another on the faded wooden benches of this 1940s train car, which must have carried so many people and seen so much over the years, Carole and I didn't mind the lack of comfort. We were enjoying the view through the weather-worn glass of the window.

Suddenly and disconcertingly, Carole's expression darkened and her face screwed up in pain. She grasped both hands to her abdomen and doubled over, seemingly in agony. I asked her what was happening, and she told me she was experiencing terrible abdominal cramps. Up until then, everything had been perfectly fine. She hadn't been experiencing any diarrhea or other intestinal symptoms at all. I didn't have any drugs with me, and my acupuncture needles were in my suitcase in the baggage compartment. What was I to do?

Carole suggested I give her a reflexology treatment. What could be simpler, I figured, and why didn't I think of that?

Reflexology is an unconventional massage technique not dissimilar to shiatsu; it involves applying pressure to specific points on the soles of the feet that correspond to the various organs in the body. It aims to improve organ function and promote relaxation and well-being. And so, sitting across from Carole, I started to gently massage the soles of her feet, focusing on the areas that correspond to the intestines. The pain faded away after five minutes, and three minutes later, she felt perfectly normal again. Was it just a coincidence, or did the treatment really work? Well, I can attest that reflexology has been very effective for my wife in this instance and on many other occasions.

Reflexology points can also be found on the outer portion of the ear, the auricle.[9] A similar technique to reflexology, **auriculotherapy** is a popular treatment in Europe[10] that was brought to light in the 1950s by Dr. Paul Nogier in the Faculty of Medicine at the University of Lyon in France. Auriculotherapy is now recognized by the World Health Organization; auriculotherapy points are also covered in acupuncture classes as they represent all the organs in the body. In some cases, patients may wear tiny needles in their outer ear to help them stop smoking or overcome drug addiction.

Although there is no scientific explanation for its effectiveness, reflexology and auriculotherapy have succeeded in helping many patients relax and relieve their pain.

Thermal treatment

The health virtues of thermal spas are often greatly extolled across the Atlantic, where many of our European cousins benefit from weeks of thermal spa treatment on medical recommendation and at public expense. I myself have visited some of these places, where the healing powers of thermal mineral water help individuals suffering from muscle and joint pain or from health conditions as varied as skin problems and pulmonary disorders. The virtues of mineral water have been known since the beginning of time, and many doctors all over Europe still prescribe these "balneotherapy" cures as therapeutic treatment strategies. Balneotherapy patients have even been found to have lower rates of anti-inflammatory drug use.[11] More than a hundred thermal spas can be found in France alone, and there are hot springs in many countries around the world. Western Canada is renowned for its hot springs, as are many U.S. states.

Hypnosis

Hypnosis is a safe, simple technique that can help to control pain. Because we all feel pain differently, the suggestions made by a hypnotherapist can modulate and diminish our perception of it. By using hypnosis, as well as altering a patient's perceived sensation of pain, I have sometimes been able to trace back and neutralize triggers in the patient's past that were causing painful chronic tension, even though the patient had forgotten all about them. This type of hypnosis is nothing like the kind you see on TV and in the movies. Medical hypnosis can benefit around 80 percent of the population, but fear often prevents people from relaxing enough to reap the benefits. People in pain can also learn some valuable self-hypnosis techniques to provide relief as and when needed. See Chapter 8 for an exercise.

Surgery

Surgery can be a key tool in dealing with chronic pain. However, it should only be used in cases where medical treatment has failed. For instance, when a case of back pain and sciatica persists and there's a danger that the sciatic nerve may be compressed for too long a time, surgical intervention will be urgently required to ensure the leg doesn't become paralyzed. The same goes in cases of pain where a conservative treatment approach fails to deliver a lasting solution. For example, a case of carpal tunnel syndrome that worsens and becomes chronic may reduce mobility in the hand and have neurological repercussions as serious as paralysis in the hand.

Some specialists may give the go-ahead for surgery right from the outset if medication is ineffective against the pain or the deterioration of an organ. With the correct diagnosis and the right surgical technique, surgery can deliver significant, beneficial, and lasting results for patients. Surgery should not be considered a last-resort solution, but a frontline treatment that has a place in every therapeutic arsenal. Surgeons' opinions are invaluable, as they're the best placed to explain to patients whether their condition warrants this kind of intervention.

AS WE'VE SEEN, there are multiple ways to ease and heal pain, and these are just some of the options out there. The World Health Organization has identified some four hundred integrative therapeutic methods around the world, and the number keeps on growing.

If something doesn't work, you don't have to give up. It's important to explore different approaches until you find the right one for you. The answers may well be different for every one of us, and I encourage you to ask questions about these various approaches to qualified professionals.

CHAPTER 7

The Psychology of Pain

The pain of yesterday is the strength of today.

PAULO COELHO

WE CAN'T TALK about pain and suffering without talking about depression. Depression can often be an unfortunate and painful—yet perfectly legitimate and common—consequence of pain, be it chronic or transitory. Regardless of its source, depression is one of our society's most widespread ills. It can be highly debilitating and is incontestably symptomatic of the times we live in. Working together, we can find solutions and bring the light at the end of the tunnel a little closer.

Pain and depression

Anyone suffering from chronic pain is likely to experience depression to some extent, and the ripple effect can easily impact on a sufferer's whole entourage. Pain can lead sufferers to scale back physical activity, rendering them vulnerable to weight gain and its ensuing health risks, which only makes matters worse. This loss of physical—and emotional—strength further increases their fragility, and there can be a tendency to retreat into isolation, aggravating the depression. In this vicious cycle, everything goes from bad to worse, because it's so easy to feel guilty, lose self-esteem, and be our own worst enemy.

Pain and its many expressions can often stir up feelings of fear. It's perfectly normal to feel worried if you don't have all the answers to what's happening to you and your body. Even if the specific cause of your pain is known, you might still be fearful if you're concerned about the long-term consequences, such as whether you'll lose your autonomy or even die prematurely, if for example you've been diagnosed with cancer. It's easy to lose hope of finding a solution, especially if you've seen several doctors and been told you have an incurable condition. You might also lose patience and get frustrated or angry at this situation you never expected to find yourself in. And most of all, you'll probably ask yourself why it's happening to you.

You might start to pull yourself together again and see hope returning little by little, but as time goes on, the hope might disappear once more and leave an opening for depression to creep in and take root. As humans, our capacity for survival is incredible—so long as we can see the light at the end of the tunnel. Individuals who can't see an end to their pain are likely to fall into depression and may compromise their very survival.

More than half of us will experience depression at some point in our lives, and that's perfectly normal. Know that these depressive states are out of our control as they affect us at a biochemical level. We'll see how later on in this chapter.

THE SYMPTOMS AND DANGERS OF DEPRESSION

If you're depressed, the main signs and symptoms you may notice include sadness, feelings of despair, loss of interest in work, distractedness, loss of productivity, weight and appetite loss, bulimic tendencies, low energy, weariness and fatigue, low libido, lack of sleep, excessive and non-restorative sleep, and crying easily or for no apparent reason. Some of these symptoms may be more obvious than others. You may also experience further ailments, such as headaches, muscle discomfort, joint stiffness, and slow digestion. To cope with these symptoms, sufferers sometimes turn to drugs or alcohol; they may easily slide into dependency and find themselves on a slippery slope toward missing days at work, financial problems, and ultimately even suicidal thoughts.

I've noticed that symptoms tend to be subtler in men than in women. Some men mistakenly think that depression is a "weakness" that men shouldn't suffer from, which means their symptoms may be expressed in different ways. For instance, increasingly frequent outbursts of impatience or anger can be signs of latent depression in men. And many may become workaholics to hide their problem. If any of this sounds familiar, it's important to ask yourself whether there's a chance you may be experiencing depression. For the sake of your work and family, depression is a possibility that shouldn't be ignored, for men and women alike.

Any thoughts of suicide, of course, should be taken very seriously. Here, again, it's important to be aware of gendered differences. Women who are experiencing suicidal thoughts tend to think about a less aggressive form of action, such as an overdose of medication, whereas men lean toward a more violent approach, such as using a firearm or a premeditated accident. Statistically, women are more likely to act on the idea, though completed suicides are more common in men. Either way, a suicide attempt is often a call for help. We shouldn't be afraid to talk about suicide with people who have depression. Simply talking about it will often relieve the pressure and help a person with depression to see hope for getting better.

TREATING BEYOND THE SYMPTOMS

Depression is an emotional state, and as a general rule, the first line of treatment involves psychological care and medication. Working with a psychotherapist is a key part of treatment, as is the ongoing care of a physician. However, it's important to bear in mind that the therapeutic response to antidepressant medication is around 50 percent. This means that 25 percent of patients will not respond at all to the medication, and 25 percent will respond randomly. What's more, the therapeutic response can be slow—it can often take three or four weeks before any relief is observed.

Medication may lead to a remission of depression, but in most cases, not to a complete recovery. Another element to add to the balance is that some studies have shown antidepressants were no more effective than placebos.[1] As with chronic illness, therefore, we must look beyond the symptoms of depression and find the cause, as well as exploring the various avenues of therapy that might get the patient back on the road to physical and psychological health. It's important to rule out any underlying health conditions that could be affecting mood, such as hypothyroidism, undiagnosed cancer, or psychological disorders. Furthermore, in cases of depression ensuing from recognized chronic pain where there the patient wasn't depressed before experiencing the pain, it's necessary to treat the individual as a whole, taking into account not only their symptoms of depression but also their physical discomfort. This is where functional medicine really comes into its own. Nothing is more satisfying for a doctor than to see a patient again who is doing much better on every level, both physically and psychologically.

THE PAIN—DEPRESSION LINK

When you're suffering, the biochemistry of pain paves the way for depression to sink its claws into you. Not many people realize this, but science is now proving that chronic pain and the inflammation it entails trigger a biochemical chain reaction that leaves you feeling depressed. The neurotransmitter disruption brought about by chronic pain can cause many patients to experience a loss of happiness and satisfaction. So don't worry if you tend to feel depressed when you're experiencing chronic pain: your neurotransmitters are the ones to blame, not you. Instead, try to accept the wave of sadness that's flowing through your body and mind.

Pain and inflammation can also change your central neurological perception so that your brain interprets pain more intensely (this is referred to as **hypersensitivity** and **hypersusceptibility** to pain). The response your brain sends to your organs will be disrupted, making the local pain more acute still. You then find yourself trapped in a vicious cycle, which your doctor has to treat as a whole before the situation can be remedied at the source. All this is more than a simple antidepressant can remedy.

Inflammation in your gut and poor-quality gut flora can also contribute to depression and can cause it to persist for longer and to a greater degree.[2] An inflamed gut will be less receptive to neurotransmitter responses, specifically to serotonin and tryptophan. Because the production and effectiveness of these "happiness" neurotransmitters is hindered, they can no longer help you.

Where stress fits in

Stress creates a lot of inflammation, and anyone who is suffering from depression will also experience some stress and anxiety. Stress can wreak havoc on all the organs in the body, even those not affected by chronic pain. When stress starts to eat away at you, it alters your very being—your cellular immunity, your general defense mechanisms, and your hormonal, digestive, and nervous systems—and your whole body pays the price.

Treating depression goes hand in hand with treating stress and the body as a whole. It's important to load up on all the good stuff, such as probiotics, prebiotics, healthy fats, omega-3s, anti-inflammatory supplements, turmeric (which works to improve inflammation and mood), B-vitamins, and vitamin D. Massage and relaxation techniques can also be beneficial. Humans are meant to be happy, and we should do everything in our power to restore the body's natural biochemistry and hit pain and depression where it hurts.

Thirty-year-old Claudia had been suffering from chronic depression for the last three years, and she was experiencing pain that never seemed to end. She wanted to come off the antidepressants she had dutifully been taking for a year to no avail, and asked for my help. Her friends told her not to worry too much, because they figured it was normal for her to feel overwhelmed and depressed by the chronic pain that had been tormenting her for so long. Claudia was experiencing pain in her neck and in the tendons in both of her shoulders. It had all started with tendinitis in her shoulders that had stemmed from her demanding work and tennis practice. She was prescribed non-steroidal anti-inflammatories (NSAIDs) for a few months, but two weeks in, the drugs started to irritate her stomach. She then started taking a Nexium-type antacid to avoid gastric ulcers.

Claudia's tendinitis pain persisted, albeit less acutely, in spite of the rest and various physiotherapy treatments she tried. However, the pain then grew generalized, and she was told there was a slight possibility she had fibromyalgia. She continued to take NSAIDs, antacids, antidepressants, and a statin because her cholesterol was too high. Shortly thereafter, she was also prescribed a sedative to help her sleep.

Claudia told me she was now so despondent she had lost all interest in her miserable life. In the questionnaire she filled out, I noticed that when she was sixteen, she had taken antibiotics for about fifteen months to treat an acne problem. Her acne had eventually gone away, only to be replaced with some intermittent, uncomfortable bloating. Then, three years ago, she had taken antibiotics again to fight two bouts of sinusitis and pneumonia.

Hearing Claudia's story, it seemed obvious to me that her digestive issue, even though the symptoms were minor, was probably the silent culprit and the source of many of her misfortunes. The bloating problem she had been experiencing for years could very well have stemmed from her prolonged use of antibiotics, which would have disrupted her entire gut flora. What's more, taking statins to reduce cholesterol levels can exacerbate muscle pain, diminish neurotransmitter quality, and affect mood.

I recommended that Claudia rebalance her gut flora by changing her diet—as suggested in Chapter 4, specifically the 5Rs approach—and adding supplements. When I saw her again four months later, she was a completely different woman. She was happy, physically active, and had lost weight. She had even gradually stopped taking her medication—under her doctor's guidance, of course. Never has the old saying by Hippocrates "Let food be thy medicine and medicine be thy food" been more true.

We know now that the gut is like a second brain in the body, where most of the neurotransmitters that are so important for our mood are produced. In Claudia's case, she likely had a neurotransmitter deficiency, hence the depression. Taking NSAIDs to ease her pain had irritated Claudia's gastrointestinal mucosa, and adding antacids to the mix had altered the pH of her flora, which led to poor absorption of vitamins and minerals. What's more, antacids deplete vitamin D, and vitamin D is a mood enhancer. In fact, Claudia's whole gut flora had been disrupted for years. She was suffering from a leaky gut (see Chapter 4) and chronic inflammation that had triggered inflammatory pain, bloating, insomnia, depression, and weight gain. So it wasn't surprising that she had had such a hard time coping.

We often see things backward: we think that because of our bad mood and depressive attitude, we've found ourselves with digestive issues and end up being diagnosed with an irritable bowel. The truth is, though, in cases like these, it's the intestinal irritability that causes the emotional irritability!

It's becoming increasingly clear that our gut shapes our emotions. And so rather than taking an antidepressant right from the outset when we have issues with depression or anxiety, it's arguably more important to take care of our gut flora and microbiota first. A defective gut will negatively affect our mood. In all likelihood, some probiotics will be seen as the antidepressants of tomorrow.

In many cases, it can be difficult to pinpoint where it all started. Was the depression caused by a leaky and inflammatory gut, or did the irritable bowel syndrome stem from the depression? Which came first, the chicken or the egg? The good news is that we can count on some strong allies to boost our morale. A healthy gut, relaxation, summer sun (in moderation), light therapy in the cold season, and neurobiofeedback or visualization, as we'll see in the next chapter, can all help to lift our mood.

Let there be light!

Seasonal depression is far more widespread than you might think, and it may affect us all at some time. When winter comes knocking at the door, the days get shorter and shorter and we start to dread the time when darkness falls mid-afternoon. The weaker the sun's rays, the fewer neurotransmitters—including serotonin, the "happiness hormone"—the body produces.

We need light. Light has a positive influence on the pineal gland, which produces melatonin and other hormones. It plays a leading role in regulating our internal body clock, which controls many functions of the body based on precise rhythms, such as our sleep-wake cycles and the secretion of various hormones at different times of the day.

After they enter the eye, light rays are converted into electrical signals, which are then sent to the brain, where they stimulate neurotransmitters. One of these is serotonin, a mood regulator that manages the production of melatonin, another hormone that controls our sleep-wake cycles. Melatonin secretion is suppressed during the daytime and stimulated at night. Hormonal irregularities caused by a lack of light can be significant enough to cause symptoms of depression.

The importance of sleep

In terms of attentiveness, presence of mind, and performance, going for nineteen hours without sleep is the equivalent of having a blood alcohol level of 0.05 percent! And it gets worse: by the same measure, going for twenty-four hours without sleep will take you over the legal drunk-driving limit.[3] As well as dulling our reflexes, a lack of sleep can make us vulnerable on many levels by lowering the body's natural defenses and depleting the nervous system.

Sleep is the time we need to recharge our batteries and repair the wear and tear in our bodies. Quality sleep is a valuable tool that helps us stay in good spirits. In today's society, with our pace of life, seven to eight hours of sleep are ideal for most of us to ensure our body and mind get the rest and recuperation they need.

When I worked a three-month stint in pediatrics, I would be on call every four days for twenty-four hours. Nights were usually busy, so most of the time I wouldn't get to close my eyes at all for those twenty-four hours. If I was lucky, I might sometimes get the chance to doze for a moment or two around five in the morning. The most obvious consequence of that schedule was that I would catch all the viral bugs that were going around, because my immune system was being stretched to the limit by all the hours of sleep I lost in the chaos of the emergency room.

Using neurobiofeedback

Your brain's health depends on its molecular components—such as vitamins, minerals, sugars, and proteins—as well as its electrical components. Brain waves are the electrical pulses produced by your brain cells to communicate with each other. In cases of depression, brain wave symmetry and location are affected, and alpha waves (the resting state for the brain), along with other types of brain waves, are disturbed. When our brain waves are out of balance, it affects mood, sleep, relaxation, attentiveness, learning in children, and even pain in general.

Neurobiofeedback is a drug-free technique that can improve brain wave patterns to counteract depression and pain. I've been exploring it for a number of years with more and more interesting results. We know today that the brain is capable of rapidly generating new neurons, and no matter how old we are, we have the capacity to produce hundreds of thousands of new brain cells.

Cardiac coherence, which we'll explore in Chapter 8, also plays an important role in neurobiofeedback because it helps boost neuron connections in the brain. Try practicing the cardiac coherence exercises on page 179, which you can do anywhere to bring your mind and body into a deep state of relaxation, promoting healing and reducing anxiety.

WHAT IS NEUROBIOFEEDBACK?

Neurobiofeedback is a form of **biofeedback**, a technique designed to help an individual gradually gain control of involuntary functions such as blood pressure, heart rate, skin temperature, and muscle tension. It uses electrodes connected to an electronic device to show the tension felt in the body on a screen. This allows the individual to become aware of this tension and try to ease it using relaxation techniques. While biofeedback is used to help mitigate the symptoms of migraine, chronic pain, post-traumatic stress disorder, and anxiety, neurobiofeedback uses electrodes placed on the scalp to view an individual's brain waves and record the brain activity on an electroencephalogram (EEG).

People suffering from anxiety, depression, or chronic pain often have brain waves that are more "scattered" than those observed in others. Neurobiofeedback uses pleasant images or sounds to reward positive brain waves, and unpleasant sounds or images to reflect negative activity. The idea is to teach the brain to work differently. Neurobiofeedback sessions, which last around half an hour, are used by some psychiatrists, psychologists, and pain specialists as a therapeutic tool for depression, anxiety, and mood disorders. After a few sessions, an EEG is typically done to monitor whether the brain waves are reorganizing in response to the treatment.

IN THE NEXT chapter we'll learn some cardiac coherence, visualization, and meditation exercises that you can use to amplify your therapeutic benefits, no matter where you are and at absolutely no cost. And we'll look at other ways to cope with pain and lessen its hold on you. By practicing these techniques, you can gain a sense of serenity and harness your physical and mental energy to foster greater well-being.

CHAPTER 8

Making Pain Easier to Live With

||||||||||||||||||||||||||||||||||||||||||||||||||||||||||||||

*Pain sometimes awakens the
strongest courage within us, and sometimes
the most vulnerable sympathy and pity.
It teaches us to stand up for ourselves and for others.*

BENJAMIN CONSTANT

S OMETIMES, NO MATTER how many doctors you see and how much you spend, no matter how hard you try and how closely you follow your treatment, it seems you just can't get rid of your pain. A number of factors might be contributing to the situation. Perhaps you still have to give it a little more time. Or maybe subconsciously, you're hanging on to the pain in some way because you feel it's your cross to bear.

Whatever the case may be, you must never lose hope. You never know when you might find a new doctor or therapist or discover a therapy you haven't tried yet. Chronic pain is something you have to explore if you want to get to the bottom of it. There might be a new therapeutic breakthrough just around the corner, or you might suddenly become aware of negative feelings that have been hindering your return to health. When pain persists against all odds, your doctor's role is to make it bearable. It's your job to use your creativity to try to turn the ordeal into a reality you can live with.

Everything that happens to us has meaning, and what we experience is a part of life. Accepting things the way they are is an art and a philosophy that can help us come to terms with our situation. We can't deny what's right in front of us, after all. Resisting and refusing to acknowledge what comes our way can only add to our pain and unhappiness. Instead of focusing on what's missing and what we've lost, we should try to be grateful for what we have.

I hope the exercises in this chapter will help to ease your pain and perhaps even eradicate it one day. Or maybe they can simply help to shift your focus and broaden your horizons so you can envision a new reality that brings hope. Perhaps this is the chance you've been waiting for to change your outlook and develop a greater awareness of who you are deep down.

Think creatively

In a way, our thoughts can help us be the architects of our lives. Thinking is the hallmark of human existence, and everything we create stems from thought.

For example, let's say you buy a new piece of furniture for your home. That object first had to be imagined by a designer, who visualized the shape, proportions, and materials, then drew up a plan before the furniture could be built. According to the principle of **creative visualization**, we must think or visualize something before it can materialize.

To be creative, the visualization we project must align with something we really think and truly believe in. This can pave the way for the abstraction we visualize to physically materialize. In my view, everything is a matter of energy. I see thought as a subtle energy that can shift and become more concrete. The more intensely and consistently we visualize something, the more tangible the results will be.

Wait, this sounds too easy and too good to be true, doesn't it? Let's not get ahead of ourselves. I'm not talking about magic; I'm talking about thinking creatively. It's not about making a fairy-tale wish, and it's certainly not about asking the universe for something we're sure we'll never get. Thinking isn't about hypocrisy or mysticism. I'll say it again: true thinking, the kind we visualize as a reality in the making, is creative.

I know skeptics will go to town with this claim, because it's something that hasn't yet been proven by medical research. I can't help but recall, though, the scientists who thought thirty-odd years ago that stress had nothing to do with the illnesses so many people suffer from today. I remember telling them back then that stress could spread quickly and make us sick, even the kind we might think is harmless because it stems from the mind. For example, imagine you have to give a presentation in a few days' time and you're worried about being judged by your peers. If, like many people, even just thinking about public speaking is enough to give you butterflies in your stomach, set your heart racing, make you sweat buckets, or tremble in fear, you might be so consumed by worry as the pressure mounts ahead of your presentation that you lose sleep for nights on end. It can even be enough to give some people a heart attack. With this in mind, is it still realistic to think that fear and stress have no impact on our health and well-being?

I chose this example to show just how creative our thoughts, beliefs, and imaginations can be, and to what extent they can shape things without us being aware. Unrelenting and involuntary thought processes can be a constant source of stress. When we fill our heads with irrational and sometimes disparaging ideas, it doesn't take much for these thoughts to sink in and for us to subconsciously create negative thought patterns that limit our perspective in life and drain our creative essence. And because these kinds of thoughts tend to be self-perpetuating, we often end up creating and experiencing the same problems in our lives over and over again.

Free yourself from toxic thoughts and guilt

In my opinion, anxiety, stress, and suppressed emotions are at the root of the majority of our ailments and pains. The influence of these negative emotions leads to changes in the autonomic (sympathetic) nervous system, immune system, and endocrine system, leaving us vulnerable to sickness or an escalation of chronic pain.[1]

Even negative thoughts can be toxic for the body. The brain is the body's pilot, and negative thoughts that disrupt the brain can dissipate toward the other organs and ultimately spread throughout the body. In a way, thoughts are the food we give to our brain. If our thoughts are distressing, our brain will suffer. If we constantly bombard our brain with negative thoughts, or if our emotions are too intense for us to handle, it's not hard to imagine the brain relieving the tension by distributing it to the other organs in the body.

In other words, I'm of the opinion that suppressed emotions will need to be expressed sooner or later as physical symptoms. There's a reason for these bodily expressions: they're the brain's way of telling us something is wrong and has to change. It may seem a little high and mighty of the brain, but when there's too much chaos going on up there, it might try to wipe its own slate clean and pass the stress on to other organs in the body, perhaps as a kind of defense mechanism.

Controlled by the nervous system, the entire endocrine system can also fall victim to these kinds of negative sentiments and cause deficiencies in the neurotransmitters—the brain proteins that dictate well-being and control pain—leading to repercussions for the body and mind. On the flip side, I strongly believe that being optimistic can have a significant positive impact on our biochemistry and help not only to keep the body in balance, but also to set us back on the road to health.[2]

Think your way out of suffering

Pain brings its share of discomfort and deprivation our way, not to mention a loss of the freedom we cherish. It demands enormous resources of patience and self-discipline—a challenging task to say the least, since pain naturally draws us into a spiral of lethargy and even depression. A little self-analysis and introspection can help us to give new meaning to this reality so we can regain control and take a new path in life.

If we know how to channel our suffering properly, we can be open to exploring a greater dimension of ourselves. How many people whose lives have been turned upside down by losing a limb, being diagnosed with cancer, or contracting a degenerative illness have transformed their suffering—and themselves—to help others in a similar position rise above their experience and rebuild a richer, happier life? There are plenty of people like this who have set an example for others to follow.

DEALING WITH THE CHALLENGE

It's not what happens to you, it's what you do about it. Our existence is based upon this principle: it's all about what we make of the events that unfold in our lives. Ultimately, we have no choice but to accept the things that happen, because they happen. We can't deny or ignore them, because they're part of our life experience. When something bad happens, we must stand *outside* of it rather than *with* it. The incident that happens *to* you is not *you*. It's important to keep a certain distance from it in your mind and avoid identifying with it directly. If what happens is a physical injury, you can acknowledge that your body is injured, but also tell yourself that you are more than that body. We are all so much more than the body we inhabit and the emotions that surge through us. Shifting our perspective so that we can become a kind of witness to what happens to us can help us cope with the minor setbacks we suffer in life and give us the strength we need to deal with any greater suffering that might come our way.

Why is it so hard to detach yourself from pain?

As we have seen, pain can certainly drive change in our lives. Curiously, we can sometimes be very accommodating of even severe and chronic pain, because it's always unsettling to detach ourselves from a situation we know well. It may seem counterintuitive, but what is familiar to us—even if it's painful—can feel safer, more reassuring, and ultimately easier than changing our habits and stepping into uncharted territory.

Anything strange and new is likely to elicit feelings of fear and insecurity and be somewhat unsettling, at least temporarily. This is why subconsciously, many of us learn to depend somewhat on our pain. We like to hold on to our beliefs and memories—the past that lies within us and makes us who we are. We live much of our lives under the influence of the past, and mistakenly believe we are the sum of all our past experiences, which prevents us from living in the present moment—the only one that is real. With this kind of attitude, not only do we cut ourselves off from the here and now; we stop the future unfolding.

Beliefs are hard to shift because they're ingrained in our deepest subconscious. Some age-old religious beliefs have long emphasized guilt by proclaiming that we are all born into sin and guilty of something right from our birth. This belief is entrenched at the deepest levels of humanity—in the Christian world, at least—and even if we're not religious, the premise can still weigh subconsciously on many of us, myself included. These deep-seated false beliefs are like weeds: they need to be completely uprooted, otherwise they'll stop any new beliefs you want to live by from taking root. If you don't face up to them and eradicate them, they will grow back again.

WHEN GUILT MAKES US SICK

We all suffer from guilt at one time or another, and some of us do every day. I remember how every time I used to go on vacation after working myself into the ground, I would get sick as soon as I stretched out on a sunny beach or set foot in a glorious green forest. Why would I get struck down by the flu or a migraine right when I was about to savor the joys of nature and enjoy some well-earned rest? Does this sound familiar to you?

I've found two possible explanations for why this happens. The first is the most Cartesian and scientific: when we're very busy and stretched to the limit, our immune system and defenses are perpetually in a high state of alert, which prevents us from getting sick, and especially from catching all sorts of flu bugs. But as soon as we release the pressure and slow down to rest and relax, our nervous and immune systems do the same, which leaves us vulnerable to all the germs around.

I had to dig deeper for the second explanation when I noticed that sometimes I got just as sick even when I hadn't worked like crazy right up until the last minute before going on vacation.

So what was causing these bouts of sinusitis and the flu that kept ruining my time off? The one to blame was still me, I realized, but it was a side of me I wasn't aware of. This other side of me had learned that he had to work hard to succeed and that there was no time for trivial things. The other me figured that vacation was a waste of time and had to punish himself if he took any time off. And so, subconsciously, I had been my own worst enemy, harboring guilt about taking too much time away. Now that I've realized this, I can properly enjoy my time away, savor the present moment, and recharge my batteries in full gratitude for the wonders of vacation.

GUILT ONLY ADDS TO YOUR SUFFERING

We must break through the psychological and mental barriers that hold us back like a ball and chain. Many of us won't achieve our full potential because once upon a time we were given a stern telling-off by our parents or put in our place by another kid at school. Our egos are fragile, and a fateful moment can become a thorn in our side for the rest of our lives. Whether it's a poor decision we made once, a humiliating experience in public, an embarrassing performance, or even just daring to stand up and say no when we "shouldn't" have, it's easy for us to chastise ourselves and feel guilt and shame. We often punish ourselves for these past experiences, even though most of the time, we can't even remember the situation that made us feel so wrong. We lose faith in our abilities, our self-confidence takes a knock, and happiness seems out of reach.

If this sounds familiar, it's time to make a change as quickly as possible. Having this kind of negative, destructive mindset will leave the people around you suffering just as much as you. Similarly, feeling guilty about your pain or thinking you're a burden for the people around you won't do any good either. Just like stress, guilt worms its way into your mind and inevitably leads to suffering. This can have a crippling effect and get in the way of you making positive changes to your life.

Learn to think bright, healing thoughts

Years of treating chronic pain have taught me that our perception can make all the difference in the intensity of the pain we feel. I sincerely believe that happiness is one of the best medicines for preserving health and reducing pain. But how can we be the picture of happiness if pain has us in its grip?

The first thing to do is to change the way we think, because thoughts have creative power. This might seem obvious, but it's easy to forget when thoughts of fear and negativity are constantly running through our minds. Since our life is shaped by our thoughts, there's no wonder it gets turned upside down and doesn't follow the course we want it to take when we think this way. These words are vitally important, so it's a good idea to reread them and put them into practice; otherwise nothing will change.

We do have a choice. We can think positive thoughts or negative thoughts, and in my mind there's no contest as to which are better. We have nothing to lose and everything to gain. We should try to formulate healthy thoughts as often as we can. To be clear, I'm not talking about being blindly optimistic and ignoring illness, or about refusing to seek help or follow appropriate treatment. It's not about fighting blindly, nor about trying to destroy sick or cancerous cells. It's about fortifying and empowering our existing healthy cells to ward off intruders.

Various approaches can help us to understand, cope with, and overcome suffering. Introspection, visualization, and meditation are all indispensable ways for us to reconnect with our deeper essence. In my opinion, having a meditation practice is a must when it comes to achieving balance and serenity. The visualization, self-hypnosis, and meditation techniques in this chapter are all vital tools that can help you get your life back on track and change it for the better.

EXERCISE 1: Controlled breathing for cardiac coherence
This controlled breathing technique is a quick and easy way to achieve **cardiac coherence**. In this state, the nervous system shifts into parasympathetic (repair and relaxation) mode. Controlled—or conscious—breathing synchronizes the breath and heart rate, which helps induce a state of relaxation throughout the organs of the body. Meditation, visualization, and prayer can also have the same effect when practiced with focus and intention.

Breathe in for five seconds, then breathe out for five seconds without holding your breath.
Repeat this ten-second breathing cycle for five minutes in total.

You can use this breathing exercise to bring about a state of cardiac coherence in just a few short minutes. Feel free to do it several times a day. This can be a good way to lead into any meditation, self-hypnosis, or visualization practice.

Using a timer can help you focus and keep your breath on track. There are a number of free apps and online videos that can help with this too (try searching "cardiac coherence" on YouTube). My favorite iOS app, RespiRelax (currently only available in French), features a rising and falling bubble—when the bubble rises, you breathe in for five seconds, and when it falls, you breathe out for five seconds. Watching the bubble helps to focus the mind and bring about the state of coherence more quickly. The app was created in conjunction with cardiac coherence specialist Dr. David O'Hare, who is considered a leading public expert in the field as well as among his peers.

Creative visualization

Creative visualization is a simple, free practice that can make a real difference in your life and for your health. As well as helping to reduce pain and stress and speed up the healing process, it can relieve and even remedy chronic conditions.[3] This technique can also help you improve your relationships with others. Elite athletes have even successfully used creative visualization to help them win competitions. Imagination and visualization are valuable tools that offer infinite possibilities, yet tend to be underused.

Any visualization involves setting yourself a goal to reach; our goal here in this chapter is to return to an optimal state of mental and physical health. This mental technique is often likened to self-hypnosis. We set our own stage on which to rid ourselves of any circumstances we no longer need and create new ones that are conducive to achieving a specific goal. By essentially reprogramming our minds to serve our well-being, we come to accept the imagined reality as an actual experience. We can tap into this creative power every day to change and enrich our daily lives.

VISUALIZATION AS COMPLEMENTARY MEDICINE

We can all make visualization a part of our lives at any time, and it won't encroach on any other kind of treatment. When I give an injection, for instance, I visualize the benefits that the substance I'm injecting will bring to the patient. I add a healing intention to my action that kicks in as soon as the substance is injected. I visualize that the patient's condition has already healed. You can apply the same principle when you take medication. Many of us are resistant to the idea of taking medication, and while I understand this point of view, because overmedication can happen, it's important not to let this kind of attitude aggravate the condition. When you're prescribed medication, don't take it begrudgingly; instead, try to visualize the good it's doing. Be mindful of the new state of health you're working toward and be grateful for the product that's transforming your body and improving your health. Allow yourself to feel the benefits the treatment is going to bring to the various parts of your body once you swallow the pill.

In the following pages, you'll find some ideas for visualization exercises. These are only a few examples, so go ahead and let your imagination run wild and create your own exercises.

You're free to write your own story, and that might well change over time. Picture yourself as the director of your own movie in your mind, and play it over and over again every day—even several times a day if you like, because the more you practice this technique, the more effective it will be. You can practice visualization anywhere, at any time, even when you're traveling for work or on vacation. Try to feed your mind these positive scenarios as much as you can; otherwise the little gremlins that fling around negative thoughts in your mind might have a field day.

Each of these exercises takes around fifteen minutes, though this might vary from person to person. Feel free to cast people you know in cameo roles in your mental movie, choose whatever location you like, and use whatever decor inspires you for your film set. If the problem is a specific health condition, find out as much as you can and familiarize yourself with the healthy morphology of the part of the body that's affected. Look up images online to help you visualize the anatomy of the area you want to nurse back to health. As well as using realistic images in your visualization, you can also bring in symbols you feel represent your personality. And remember, your attitude is important: you must be confident in what and who you are, as well as what you feel.

Imagine you've already achieved your goal. And no matter what story you project, always be gentle with yourself and do these exercises with love and intention.

Have you tried visualization and you still can't see anything? Don't worry. Focus on feeling deep down what and who you are. Let that feeling spread within you, and the benefits will be just as great.

VISUALIZATION AND SELF-HYPNOSIS

Self-hypnosis is a technique that can be used in conjunction with visualization, before projecting the images and while projecting them. This technique is similar to hypnosis, in that it relaxes the mind and brings the individual to a state of great peace. We call this an induction phase, in which the conscious mind gives in to the subconscious mind. Outside help—typically from the hypnotist—is generally required for the individual to enter this state. In self-hypnosis, however, the individual induces the altered state of consciousness alone, in a very gentle, natural way. This process can then be a gateway to amplify the power of the visualization that follows. Ideally, we would always use self-hypnosis and visualization side by side.

You can stream free audio recordings of the following exercises from my website at drbrouillard.com.

EXERCISE 2: Self-hypnosis

This self-hypnosis exercise will guide you gently and safely into a beneficial state of relaxation. You will find this technique invaluable before any visualization or meditation as it will help to bring about the peace of mind we're all seeking. Feel free to use this technique as often as you like. Resting your mind and freeing it from the pressures of everyday life will automatically lead your body into a state of relaxation and unlock its full creative power.

Sit comfortably with your legs uncrossed and your feet on the floor, or in the lotus position if you prefer.

Close your eyes and exhale deeply, very deeply.

Now inhale slowly, deeply, drawing the air deep into your belly and allowing it to expand fully.

Exhale gently, deeply, and let all the air out of your rib cage and belly completely.

Follow this breathing pattern calmly three times.

Turn your awareness to the crown of your head.

Feel your scalp relax. Feel it sending gentle waves of calm through your head and your mind. Feel these gentle waves of relaxation as they wash over your eyelids.

Your eyelids are feeling heavier and heavier, more and more relaxed.

You feel happy and contented.

Send your awareness to your eyes.

The muscles of your eyes are relaxed.

Send your awareness to your jaw.

Your jaw is becoming more and more relaxed; you are feeling more and more relaxed as the wave of relaxation slowly washes over your body . . . your neck . . . your shoulders . . . your chest.

Your breathing is calm and peaceful.

Feel this wave of relaxation and peace wash slowly over your whole body.

Relax your belly . . . your hips . . . your legs.

Your legs are feeling more and more relaxed and rested.

Feel the lightness in your legs.

Feel this wave of relaxation wash all the way down to your feet, to the tips of your toes.

You feel wonderful, perfectly relaxed, from the crown of your head to the tips of your toes.

A wave of tranquility flows through your whole body.

You are savoring this moment of peace and well-being.

Now visualize a ball of energy at your feet, a ball of blue light— beautiful blue light.

This blue ball of light is going to bring more and more calm to your body.

Visualize the ball as it rolls between your ankles, rolling away any residual tension.

As the ball rolls up your legs, your legs feel so light and relaxed.

The ball keeps on rolling, over your hips, into your belly, into your chest.

Feel how much easier it is to breathe now that you are so light and relaxed.

This beautiful blue ball of light is filling your lungs and lifting your heart.

Feel the calm, relaxing effect of this shining ball of light.

Let the ball roll up over your neck, into your head.

Let it fill your mind with light; let it fill you with peace and serenity.

Enjoy this moment of relaxation that you have chosen to offer yourself.

Now you're ready to try the next exercise (or any other visualization exercise you feel like treating yourself to).

EXERCISE 3: Your inner smile (visualization)

The following exercise can induce a profound sense of calm and harmony and promote gland regeneration. Hormones are secreted in your body under the guidance of a well-oiled nervous system and a cool, calm, and collected mind. Your glands are the masterminds of your body, and they can work in harmony when you fill them with goodness and serenity.

To ensure you get the most out of this visualization, I suggest you look at the following illustration, as it will help you to picture how these glands work inside your body.

Major glands

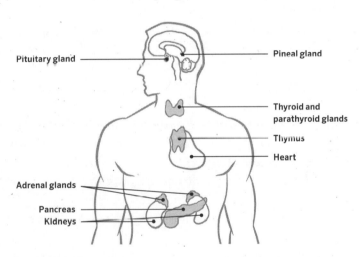

The **pineal gland** is located in the center of your head. It's about the size of a pea, and some say it is the seat of the soul. It secretes the key hormone melatonin, which regulates your sleep and wake cycles. Melatonin is known as the hormone of youth, as it also protects your DNA and immune system.

The **pituitary gland** is located just in front of the pineal gland, between your eyes. It coordinates all the other glands farther down your body to keep them working in harmony.

The **thyroid gland** converts iodine into thyroid hormones to generate the lifeblood of your being and drive your mental creativity.

Your **thymus** plays a protective role by strengthening your entire immune system.

The **adrenal glands** are two little glands perched on top of your **kidneys** that help keep you strong through times of physical and emotional stress. They too need to be calm and rested to make sure all your organs get the downtime they need.

At the crown of your head, visualize a happy smile filled with calm, contentment, and serenity.

This sweet smile spreads slowly, gently down from the crown of your head to your soft lips.

You feel good, you feel relaxed and fully present in this smile.

Now visualize a moment in your life when everything was relaxed and easy.

Perhaps you were walking through a field in the countryside without a care in the world.

Feel this moment of calm happiness right at the center of your head, in your pineal gland. This gland is the gateway to your spiritual being. Feel how this place is a haven of tranquility.

Imprint a smile of contentment and well-being on your pineal gland.

Now take this smile and extend it to your pituitary gland, right between your eyes.

Feel the gentle tingling, a sense of delight sparkling between your eyebrows.

These two glands are reveling in joy and tranquility.

The smile keeps growing and moves down to kiss your lips.

Now it moves down to your throat and spreads the love into your thyroid gland, giving you more and more vitality.

Feel the lightness here.

Your thyroid gland has two lobes, and these lobes are like the wings of a butterfly, a silky, light butterfly that's ready to fly away and leave all the noise and busyness behind.

Now you feel this smile spreading down into your thymus, just above the level of your heart.

Now the smile is right at the center of your body, at the very heart of your being, the heart that pulses life into each and every one of your cells.

Your heart is much more than a pump to move blood around your body; it's your lifelong friend, a little brain that beats tirelessly in time to your emotions and breathes life into your cells from your head to your toes.

Thank your heart warmly with this joyful smile.

Now keep spreading the smile down into your solar plexus.

Flood your liver and spleen with the light from this glowing smile.

Keep going, down to the tops of your kidneys, and thank both of your adrenal glands for keeping you safe from infection and protecting you from the stresses of life itself. They give you strength, stability, and warmth. Your smile brings them comfort and strength in turn.

Feel the smile spread down toward your reproductive organs and gently embrace these wonderful creators of life.

Now feel your smile lifting all the way back up to your brain, ready to connect to your entire nervous system.

Guide the smile down the great vagus nerve that runs from your brain all the way down through your abdomen. You are nourishing your parasympathetic nervous system, which helps you to relax and helps all your cells to regenerate.

This smile of goodness is now touching every part of your body, from the crown of your head to the tips of your toes.

Allow yourself to enjoy this state of calm for about five minutes while the smile works all its magic.

Now thank your body for welcoming this wonderful smile and for working so hard to regenerate so much, over and over again.

EXERCISE 4: The triangle of peace, harmony, and love (visualization)[4]
This is a simple but oh-so-beneficial exercise that works wonders when you make a good habit of doing it regularly. It's all about using the force of the triangle formed by three very important glands—the pineal, the pituitary, and the heart—which work in harmony to keep us in balance. When you do this exercise every day with intention, you'll be surprised by the results in your body and mind. Think of it like taking a daily vitamin: the effects are barely noticeable the first week, but over the weeks and months that follow, your biochemistry will improve and your whole being will feel the benefits.

It's important to be familiar with controlled breathing technique before you start this exercise. It builds on the cardiac coherence technique we saw in Exercise 1 (page 179), which quickly brings the body into a state of physiological, mental, and emotional balance.

The triangle of peace, harmony, and love

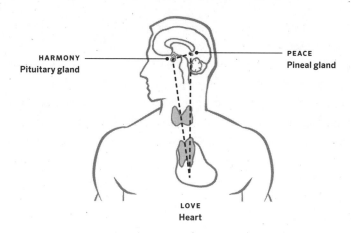

HARMONY
Pituitary gland

PEACE
Pineal gland

LOVE
Heart

Sit comfortably with your feet on the floor, or sit in the lotus position.
Take three deep breaths.
Every breath you take brings you deeper into relaxation than the last.
Breathe slowly, deeply.

Now bring yourself into a state of cardiac coherence by using the technique we saw earlier: six breaths a minute for five minutes.

Focus your awareness on the pineal gland. This little gland is right at the center of your head. This is your connection to the whole universe.

Breathe the word PEACE into this place; feel the peace flowing through this gland and throughout your head. Allow peace to settle in calmly, deep inside this little gland in your head.

Feel the sense of contentment and well-being it gives you.

Now turn your awareness to your pituitary gland. It's right there between your eyes.

This is the master gland, the conductor of the whole orchestra of other glands in the body.

It's the hub that connects all your cells and glands.

Breathe the word HARMONY into your pituitary gland.

Deep inside, feel the wellness and synchronicity this gland gives to you.

Turn your awareness down toward your heart. Your heart does much more than pump blood around your body; it's a gland filled with intelligent neurons. It's the brain at the center of your body.

It's like a computer that processes your every reaction.

Your heart gland has an incredible magnetic power that radiates out in constant communication with your inner world and the world around you.

Not even the slightest pressure can escape it.

Give it all of your love.

Breathe the word LOVE into this compassionate heart of yours.

Feel the love pulsing and radiating through your body and out into the world around you.

Thank your heart for all the tireless work it does.

Now repeat within yourself with conviction, appreciation, and determination, these three words—Peace, Harmony, Love—as you visualize the triangle formed by your pineal gland, your pituitary gland, and your heart.

Repeat these three words three times in your mind or out loud as you visualize your triangle—from the center of your head to the point between your eyes and down to your heart in your chest.

When you reach your heart, pause for a moment to feel the love radiating out from there before moving back up to complete the triangle and start again: Peace, Harmony, Love.

You can also do this exercise with these words in the same order: LIGHT – STRENGTH – LOVE.

To imprint this peace, harmony, and love even deeper in your being, you can try placing your hands over your heart and pressing lightly as you visualize each of these three words and places.

Meditation

Meditation offers us a way to detach ourselves from the pain that is weighing us down like an anchor. It brings us into a space where we can step back and see ourselves as being more than just our pain—the pain that is consuming our lives, preoccupying us, sometimes to the point of making us want to shut out our loved ones and everything around us.

Meditation is a spiritual practice, but it's not a religion. The famous philosopher René Descartes once argued that there were two realities: material reality and spiritual reality. I imagine spiritual reality as this consciousness, this higher intelligence, this soul we all have within us, whether we're aware of it or not.

With many of us leading such hectic lives and often feeling restless and scattered, it's becoming increasingly important for us to make time to simply reflect, focus, and retreat into ourselves. When we slow and calm our thoughts, we reconnect with our deepest essence. It's about *being* rather than doing or having—simply being present and accepting what comes along. Cultivating this state of mind lets us detach ourselves from our suffering, and meditation is one way for us to do this.[5]

I can never stress enough how important it is to develop a daily meditation practice, and by this I mean meditating about what's happening around us and what we're feeling inside. Meditation is a daily need, just like the food we eat. Meditation is food for the soul, which we must nourish every day to stay connected to our true values and keep stress at bay. Even if we feel pressed for time, it's important to take at least ten minutes for ourselves every day. This can make all the difference, not only for the day ahead, but also for the rest of our lives.

There are many ways and reasons to meditate. One is to reduce pain—or acknowledge its ultimate source—by shifting our attention away from the painful area. To enter a state of meditation, we must calm the body and mind; for this it's essential to find and stay in a comfortable position and focus on the rhythm of the breath.

Conscious breathing is an important part of meditating (see Exercise 1). Starting your meditation practice with this conscious breathing exercise will quickly reduce the intensity of the pain you're feeling, too. Once you've done five minutes of conscious breathing, you're ready to start the meditation of your choice. The many scientific benefits of meditation are still being discovered. On a spiritual level, meditation can help us reconnect to our deepest inner beings and ultimately may give us some answers to why we are suffering.

WHAT IF I FEEL TOO STRESSED TO MEDITATE?

If you're extremely stressed or find yourself in an exceptionally uncomfortable situation and feel overwhelmed, you may feel so jittery and on edge that the very idea of sitting down to relax, gather your thoughts, and meditate might seem impossible. When your heart's pounding in your chest and waves of emotions keep flooding over you, it's easy to tell yourself that it's all your fault and that you're making things worse.

What's happening is perfectly normal, however: your adrenaline and cortisol levels are spiking and throwing your body and mind off balance. Before you can do anything else, you have to reduce this hormonal toxicity.

Vigorous exercise can help to dissipate and burn off these hormones. Think about the fight-or-flight response that kicks in when an animal feels threatened by a predator and runs away as fast as it can. Sometimes your mind can be the predator and hunt you down when you're standing dead still! Once you've had a good workout and your cortisol and adrenaline levels have returned to normal, you'll find it easier to relax. What's more, exercise promotes the secretion of beneficial hormones and neurotransmitters to further enhance well-being. That's another good reason to get some exercise!

For some people, a more active and dynamic form of meditation may work better. One way to do this might be to go for a run in the woods and be mindful of your surroundings and state of mind. Others may find listening to music and moving their body in a free, spontaneous way more effective for them. Natural movement can be a great way for us to loosen up both body and mind. Let's not forget either that we humans are constantly evolving, and that not all forms of traditional meditation will suit everyone. There's always room for new techniques to evolve—and keep us evolving too!

EXERCISE 5: *Tonglen* (compassionate meditation) to alleviate suffering
This technique can help to develop compassion by embracing the suffering of others as part of our own meditation. The well-being we can bring to those around us is surely the best present we can give, not only to the other person, but also to ourselves. Have you ever heard the saying that it's by giving that we receive the most?

This very simple technique dates back to the year 1000 and is attributed to the Indian sage Atisha. His Holiness the fourteenth Dalai

Lama is said to practice this meditation every day. I took the opportunity to familiarize myself with the altruistic technique of *Tonglen*—a word that means giving and receiving—more than twenty years ago under the aegis of Etbonan Karta, and I have certainly appreciated the benefits. This meditation helps us to absorb what is negative, process it, and breathe it back out into the world as positive. What makes this technique so interesting is that instead of asking for relief from our own hardship, we bring the suffering of others into ourselves and turn it into positive thoughts so that we can restore peace and loving kindness to others, thus relieving their pain.

Regular practice of this meditation will allow us to overcome our fears and accept events that happen outside ourselves. It will help us to move beyond criticism and judgment of the world and of others, and lead us to accept what is before us as a simple fact. The first few times, I suggest you do this meditation for yourself. When you feel calm and confident enough, then you can try the original version and meditate for others.

Let's begin.

Sit comfortably with a straight back. Breathe slowly, calmly. In your mind, pick a negative feeling that is weighing on your mind, a pain that is nagging at you, a fear, something you are angry about, or anything else that is bothering you.

Close your eyes and take three deep breaths to calm your mind. With every breath, feel a sense of calm fill your body. As you grow calmer and calmer, you feel the flow of your thoughts start to slow down. You are becoming more and more present within yourself. Every breath relaxes you a little more. You are calm and collected.

Now, as you keep breathing normally, turn your awareness to the feeling you wanted to get rid of, the feeling that is preventing you from being yourself, from being happy and at peace; pick it up and put it down in front of you. Stay focused on your breathing and on this feeling.

Imagine this tension and suffering is a cloud of smoke right in front of you. Start to breathe this smoke into your body with confidence. See the cloud getting smaller as you draw this smoke into your body and imagine it turning into a bright light that shines deep inside your being. As the smoke disappears, there is only light within you. Breathe out joy, love, courage, strength, peace, or whatever feels the most positive for you.

Visualize the same negative feeling again as smoke and breathe it in. As the smoke disappears, it lights a flame within you. Now breathe this out as joy, love, courage, strength, peace, or whatever feels the most positive for you.

Repeat this exercise several times with every breath you take.

When you're comfortable with the technique, feel free to try the traditional altruistic version of this meditation to develop compassion for another person. This person may be your child, your partner, a friend, someone you know who is suffering, or someone you rarely see anymore because they have somehow offended you.

You can also choose to dedicate this meditation to the polluted environment, a humanitarian crisis, or even a politician to help bring about a more compassionate, enlightened form of governance. There's no shortage of people or causes to meditate for, so do whatever you feel is important for you and for the greater good.

The opportunity of pain

Pain can be an opportunity for us to step back and reflect deep down on our kindness toward ourselves and others. Extinguishing pain— or at least making it easier to live with—by changing the way we approach it can bring out some wonderful qualities within ourselves that we weren't even aware of.

This inner search, imbued with goodness and compassion, is like a healing balm for the pain we're struggling through. For it to penetrate deep down beneath our skin, we have to look beyond the pain we're feeling in a given part of the body. Without judging, let's allow ourselves to simply observe moments of pain and irritation, bringing to them a new vision and direction that will make our lives richer and better. Now that we know some of the basics, it's up to us what we do with this knowledge.

THE POWER OF FORGIVENESS

A chronic physical pain that digs in its heels and persists in spite of appropriate treatment may have been generated by old grudges toward ourselves or others that we may have been carrying around for so long we've forgotten them. If we force ourselves to turn the page, we can finally rid ourselves of this painful burden and feel lighter and freer.

Forgiveness is a form of relief that can renew our zest for life as well as freeing the tension that resentment, anger, and bitterness can cause. It's not about forgetting; it's about sincerely forgiving. True forgiveness allows us to release the toxic feelings that can lead to unexplained headaches, recurring muscle pain, irritability, anxiety, and even depression.[6] Forgiveness can be an effective painkiller for both the person receiving it and the person giving it.

Who doesn't have something—or someone—to forgive? It might be an absent parent, an abusive experience in childhood, a painful separation, or a betrayal of trust. Whatever or whoever we have to forgive, we must first acknowledge the pain we're feeling in different parts of our body and mind, and not try to forget it. We must be able to feel it before we can forgive and finally feel relief.

I remember seeing a documentary once about the Vietnam War and John Plummer, the man who claimed to be the U.S. pilot who bombarded a Vietnamese village with the burning gas napalm. An iconic photo taken in 1972 that made the cover of Life *magazine at the time had shown a poor nine-year-old girl by the name of Kim Phúc with burns to more than*

60 percent of her naked body, fleeing the flames consuming a Buddhist temple where her family had taken refuge from the American bombings. After fourteen months in hospital and at least seventeen surgical procedures, Kim finally returned home. She tried to lead a normal life again and go on to medical school, but the Vietnamese government soon tracked her down and forced her to interrupt her studies to make her a poster child denouncing the atrocities of the Vietnam War.

Resisting this authoritarian directive, she sought asylum in Canada during a trip to Newfoundland in 1992. Despite her young age, she knew very well that dwelling on the horrors and suffering of her past would only make things worse and stop the pain from disappearing. She had already moved on to a more positive life, leaving the atrocities and ugliness of the war behind her. Forgiveness had already started to work its magic on her. The healing process was going well and the pain was gradually beginning to wane. In spite of all the suffering from her burns and various operations, her whole being radiated beauty, goodness, and a zest for life, as if the painful scars of the past had faded.

Years later, at a ceremony in Washington commemorating the Vietnam War, Kim Phúc gave a moving speech about world peace. "Even if I could talk face to face with the pilot who dropped the bombs, I would tell him we cannot change history, but we should try to do good things for the present and for the future to promote peace," she said. As it happened, John Plummer, whose soul had been ravaged by the war, was there in the crowd. Moved by her message of peace and love, he passed a note to her on a scrap of paper saying that he was the man who had dropped the bombs on the temple and her village.

Leaving her microphone behind, she ran right over to Plummer with open arms and hugged him. Sobbing, he told her he was sorry, and she replied that everything was okay and that she had forgiven him a long time ago. From that point on, the nightmares and pain that had been plaguing Plummer for twenty-five years disappeared. The ex-serviceman felt relieved of a huge weight and went on the become a pastor in the year that followed. He later admitted that he was not in fact the pilot who had dropped the bombs on the village and the temple, nor was he the man who had ordered the attack. However, he explained that he had felt terribly guilty because he was serving in the U.S. Army in Vietnam during the war, and that he had passed the note during the ceremony because he had been overcome by emotion. Phan Thi Kim Phúc now lives near Toronto and is a UNESCO *Goodwill Ambassador.*

Forgiveness is a mental exercise that we can all do ourselves. You can do this practice of intention and compassion even without the other person being there. Sit comfortably and think about a situation that bothered you. Replay the situation in your mind with a calm, detached attitude, as if you were a witness to this situation, watching a movie with an actor playing your role. Being a witness in this way helps to quell any volatile emotions that come up for you. Now visualize that scene again with a clearer head and greater understanding for the person who hurt you. Try to accept it as something that happened and is now in the past. It no longer belongs to you and you can let it go.

To break free of the shackles of this pain, it's important to detach yourself from the situation. You have to set aside any notions of good, bad, and guilt. Forgiveness is an act of inner peace that frees the body, mind, and spirit and benefits your entire being. It's a formative and transformative experience that's not just liberating for you, but also unknowingly for the person you are forgiving.

GRATITUDE COSTS NOTHING

Gratitude is recognition; it's a feeling of happiness with what we have and what we can become. It can relieve stress and enhance our well-being.[7] Saying thank you is just the tip of the iceberg—gratitude is something we must feel in the here and now and make a part of our everyday lives. It's a gateway to health and happiness, and it can change your life. All you have to do is acknowledge what you have received and recognize what life gives you, day in, day out—be that simply the experience of living, or perhaps an ailment that's troubling you and making you realize how precious your health is. We all feel gratitude from time to time, but it's an easy sentiment to forget because we soon fall back into old habits and revert to what we know. We tend to take the gift of life and the people around us for granted.

⁜⁜⁜⁜⁜⁜⁜⁜⁜⁜⁜⁜⁜⁜⁜⁜⁜⁜⁜⁜⁜⁜⁜⁜⁜

EVEN IF YOU'RE in pain, gratitude can give you a positive outlook on life. Even better, it can help you be present and mindful of what's right before your eyes. Invariably, you can detach yourself from your past by developing an ever-present sense of gratitude. There's no place for self-pity anymore, no matter how intense your pain may be. Contemplate every moment and be mindful that it is unique. Acknowledge that you are a part of the present moment. We all have a unique and important role to play in life. Life is constantly giving us signs and trying to awaken us to something greater. Let's be mindful of the gift we are given every single minute of our lives. Every step we take can be a miracle if we truly understand the impact it can have.

Conclusion

||||||||||||||||||||||||||||||||||||||||||||||||||||||||||||||||||||||||||||

'VE BEEN EXPLORING pain for so long, it feels like an old friend. In this book, I've tried to explain the many aspects of pain and shed some light on the very real conditions I treat. Pain is an opportunity for us to recognize an imbalance in the body. It sounds the alarm to let us know there's a problem to fix. Even though pain is always bothersome and sometimes incapacitating, I wanted to show you how that same pain can be the starting point for positive change, be it a change to your lifestyle, environment, or way of thinking.

Understandably, our first reflex is often to try to silence the pain and revert to some external means, such as medication or physical treatment, in an attempt to get back to our routine and put the inconvenience behind us as quickly as possible. However, I think it's important to encourage ourselves to dig a little deeper and expose the often-overlooked causes of some frequent ailments, as well as the more common triggers. I also wanted to open your eyes to some lesser-known treatments that have brought relief to many of my patients, sometimes permanently. We also explored the psychological factors that can give rise to pain and affect our relationship with suffering. Finally, how could I not touch on the incredible power of the mind to help us live with pain in our daily lives?

THE TIME FOR TREATMENT IS NOW

If we want to bring an end to our pain—which can turn into suffering if it seeps deep down into our being—we must accept that no matter what happens, life has placed this obstacle in our path for us to overcome. Treating our pain starts where we are right now, by reading this book and bringing the principles it contains into our lives from this moment on. Life is one big game, and we must play our best on the board we're given. We must stay positive and play fair no matter how frustrated we get. We can't deny, refuse, or ignore this life.

Being human means suffering sometimes, and accepting this is the first step toward freeing ourselves from that suffering. We must accept things as they are and accept who we are—we won't be true to ourselves otherwise. We must admit that we're vulnerable and be honest with the facts life brings our way. Instead of trying to find the meaning of life, it's up to us to bring meaning to our lives!

I like to think that we are all explorers on this planet and have a duty to keep scaling new heights rather than giving up when obstacles stand in our way. Let's at least hope that for every step we take on our quest to ease our pain, we gain more experience and become a little calmer, a little wiser, and a little more enlightened.

The way we react to pain is crucial and can have a huge impact on our quality of life. There's no point blaming ourselves for what's happening to us or for the suffering we've caused to ourselves or to others. We must learn to tackle new and challenging situations with confidence, empathy, and detachment. These are the attitudes that will keep us from falling into the trap of suffering.

Everything we see, everything we hear, and everything we touch is there for us to feel our presence in the universe. Being consciously present and appreciating what's right in front of us will keep sadness, depression, and pain at bay. The pain won't necessarily disappear, but something greater will emerge—a feeling of being a part of the grand scheme of life, in all our wonderful uniqueness.

Pain Guide

||||||||||||||||||||||||||||||||||||||||||||||||||||||||||||||

I N THIS BOOK, we've explored various options for rethinking pain and all its physical and psychological implications. This appendix can serve as a reference guide for pain in the body from head to toe. It's designed to help you understand the causes of many common conditions. You'll also find some practical tips for overcoming your pain more quickly. Obviously, these therapeutic solutions aren't here to stop you from putting into practice what you learned earlier in this book. When all is said and done, knowing the hows and whys of your pain and making the right lifestyle choices is always good for your health.

Pain from head to toe

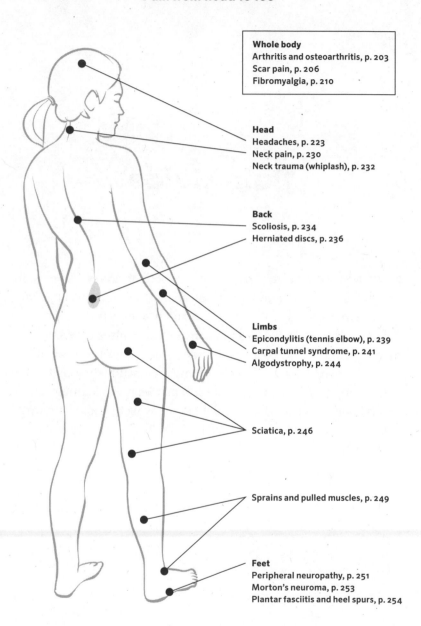

Whole body
Arthritis and osteoarthritis, p. 203
Scar pain, p. 206
Fibromyalgia, p. 210

Head
Headaches, p. 223
Neck pain, p. 230
Neck trauma (whiplash), p. 232

Back
Scoliosis, p. 234
Herniated discs, p. 236

Limbs
Epicondylitis (tennis elbow), p. 239
Carpal tunnel syndrome, p. 241
Algodystrophy, p. 244

Sciatica, p. 246

Sprains and pulled muscles, p. 249

Feet
Peripheral neuropathy, p. 251
Morton's neuroma, p. 253
Plantar fasciitis and heel spurs, p. 254

Arthritis and osteoarthritis

Arthritis and osteoarthritis are a source of constant pain for sufferers. Pain ends up being a fact of life for them, as disconcerting as that can be. While these conditions often begin to set in as we grow older, more and more frequently, even relatively young people are finding themselves affected.

Arthritis and osteoarthritis are two separate conditions, but they can trigger similar symptoms, which is why we're looking at them together in this section. Both cause the kind of joint pain we generally refer to as rheumatism.

ARTHRITIS

Arthritis is a general term used to describe inflammation in the joints (the "itis" suffix means inflammation). The four cardinal signs of inflammation are pain, heat, redness, and swelling. The inflammatory nature of arthritis makes it an "active," or progressive, disease that will tend to deform the joints over time. **Rheumatoid arthritis** is a common type of arthritis that affects and inflames entire joints. This means it can extend to the ligaments, joint capsules, tendons, and occasionally other parts of the body, such as the heart and eyes. Even the skin can be affected by a form of arthritis, known as **psoriatic arthritis**. The pain of arthritis is aggravated by prolonged periods of rest—such as a night of sleep—to the point where the swelling can even cause the joint to lock up. Some gentle movement (limbering up in the morning) can help to alleviate the pain.

Arthritis tends to affect major joints, such as the knees, hips, and shoulders, though it can affect many other joints as well. Certain forms of arthritis may affect the lumbar vertebrae or sacroiliac joints. One example is **ankylosing spondylitis**, which can manifest in patients in their twenties, causing pain and stiffness in the back. Some rare, but much more serious, types of arthritis may be triggered by an infection and will often affect the whole body and cause a fever.

Rheumatoid arthritis is certainly the most common form of arthritis, and it's one of the autoimmune diseases that are growing increasingly frequent today. When the symptoms first begin, it can be difficult to distinguish rheumatoid arthritis from osteoarthritis. However, the treatment for each of these conditions will be very different because of their severity, the extent of the lesions, and especially their origin. Breathing polluted air and eating processed food lacking in nutrients are both contributing to the growing incidence of this condition.

Leaky gut syndrome (see Chapter 4 on intestinal permeability) is often a precursor to arthritis and a warning that we should address predisposing factors, which include toxins, harmful gut bacteria, stress, and food intolerances.[1] The 5Rs approach covered in Chapter 4 can help patients to break free from this form of arthritis.

TREATMENT OPTIONS

Standard pharmaceutical treatments for arthritis are mainly non-steroidal anti-inflammatory drugs (NSAIDs), steroids such as cortisone, antineoplastics (anti-cancer drugs used in chemotherapy), and TNF (tumor necrosis factor) inhibitors. However, all of these powerful drugs can cause devastating side effects and will not cure the disease itself, thus influencing its progression. It's important for your doctor to look at the big picture and first address the source of the problem. With autoimmune diseases, it's more important to ask *why* the person is developing antibodies that are attacking the body's own cells; treating the person's symptoms is only a partial solution.

OSTEOARTHRITIS

Osteoarthritis is a degenerative joint condition. Just like rust attacks old metal hinges, osteoarthritis causes the mechanical workings of our joints to seize up, usually when we reach old age. Osteoarthritis causes the cartilage of the joints to wear and break down. It tends to affect mainly the fingers, feet, hips, knees, and back as we get older. However, it's not uncommon for young people who practice so-called extreme sports to develop osteoarthritis as a result of repetitive injuries to the knees and spine, for example.

Osteoarthritis is mainly diagnosed by X-ray. Unfortunately, this may not be the most reliable indicator. All too often, joint pain is labeled as osteoarthritis as soon as an X-ray shows signs that might suggest the condition. However, many patients present clear radiological signs of osteoarthritis without feeling the slightest pain. On the flip side, around 10 percent of patients feel significant pain in their joints despite only minimal signs of osteoarthritis on their X-rays. Even MRIs struggle to yield further clues that might explain this intense pain.

We used to think that the more the cartilage wore away, the more the joint would hurt, but this bone-on-bone theory is now somewhat outdated. Just because the joint has suffered a significant loss of cartilage, it doesn't mean it will be very painful. The inflammation in the joint actually generates more pain than the mechanics of the joint itself.

In all cases of osteoarthritis, it's important to pinpoint the neurological dysfunction that is triggering the pain, which may be cerebral or local. Hypersensitivity will be caused by the inflammation that is partially destroying the joint, ligament, tendons, or synovial capsule. Every patient and their perception of pain are unique (as with fibromyalgia), and the underlying causes of osteoarthritis can be just as numerous.

TREATMENT OPTIONS

Osteoarthritis calls for a multifaceted treatment approach to address the various dysfunctional aspects or systems of the individual patient. In other words, because osteoarthritis pain is more than just a local problem in the joint, we must treat the person as a whole. Some supplements (see Chapter 5) may be useful for their anti-inflammatory properties, including glucosamine, chondroitin, MSM (methylsulphonylmethane, which promotes collagen production), and proteolytic enzymes. In some cases, anti-inflammatory drugs may be used as complementary treatment, and injections may be effective.

Scar pain

When you injure yourself or have surgery, it's normal for there to be a scar. Scars are an unfortunate fact of life and can stay with us forever, even if surgeons take every precaution to keep them as discreet as possible. But are scars harmless? Some never lead to any consequences, but most will, to some extent. When a scar heals, some adhesions inevitably form around the area. It becomes an attachment point for the surrounding tissue, including the fascia (muscle envelopes). This can often generate pain and discomfort, including referred pain, even if there is no pain path leading from the scar itself.[2]

Unexplained chronic pain is commonly found to be caused by a scar—an association that many of us would never have suspected. Scar pain is a frequent cause for consultation at pain clinics and affects thousands of individuals, sometimes for years on end. The more surgeries an individual has, the greater the risk of scar pain developing. For this reason, we should pay careful attention to scars and consider desensitizing them using the techniques outlined below. Even small, superficial scars deserve a closer look, in my opinion.

Bigger, deeper scars, of course, will usually form adhesions in the body. These fibrous bands, made of multiple filaments woven like a spider's web, form after any incision or surgery and can create tension in the surrounding organs. The more invasive the surgery, the greater the risk of adhesions, and they're especially common with abdominal surgery. I see many patients who are experiencing pain five years or more after having abdominal surgery, and no one has ever thought to take a look at their belly!

The pain caused by a scar can present in various ways. You may experience itching, a burning sensation, or a stabbing pain. This kind of pain can become unbearable and severely hinder a patient's daily activities. On top of the fibrosis and pulling on the surrounding tissue, the scar can also cause nerve damage and generate neuropathic pain, which manifests not only around the scar itself but also in the areas up and down the nerve paths. For example, there may be pain not only in the lumbar spine, but also in the buttocks and sometimes even down one leg. Often, this kind of pain responds very reluctantly to painkillers and anti-inflammatories.

In cases of unexplained abdominal pain where tests have come back negative, an abdominal examination is in order. Palpating the abdomen can detect any adhesions that may be generating local or even referred pain. A healthy abdomen shouldn't be sensitive to palpation or have any areas of hardness. Problematic scars may predispose individuals to vague digestive issues, back pain, and even chest pain.

In women, the relationship between adhesions and pelvic pain remains unclear. We do know, however, that adhesions cause pain. And in all likelihood, they hinder organ mobility, leading to pulling and discomfort, and impact the nerves themselves. It's not uncommon for women who have undergone gynecological abdominal surgery to complain of pain in the perineum, even though the surgery was performed much farther up the body. The same effects can sometimes be observed after a C-section.

Mastectomy is one surgical procedure that can leave particularly significant scars. Breast tissue is highly sensitive in both women and men. One of my patients, who was suffering from gynecomastia (hormonal swelling of male breast tissue), had undergone a double mastectomy. His scars were as visible as they were painful, but the pain went away after a few sessions of treatment.

Sternotomy—a major surgical procedure used in open-heart surgery that involves opening the sternum—can also open the door to a similar kind of pain.

I remember one patient who consulted with me two years after undergoing open-heart surgery, for chest pain that was radiating into his shoulders and ribs. He had talked to his surgeon about it, worried that his heart problems might be coming back. His surgeon told him that his heart was healthy and he had nothing to worry about. He was prescribed painkillers and anti-inflammatories. However, the intense pain persisted and was preventing the patient from functioning.

Upon examination, I couldn't help but notice a scar on the patient's sternum that must have been seven inches long. The scar was still thick, despite the time that had gone by, and decidedly painful along its whole length. The area of the ribs attached to the sternum, around the scar, was also very sensitive. I explained to the patient that his scar might well be to blame for the pain he was feeling every day. I suggested a number of xylocaine injections to desensitize the area, with a little cortisone to reduce the swelling and thickness. The patient felt considerable relief from the pain within minutes of the very first injection, and even found he had less difficulty breathing. After four visits over a two-month period, the patient experienced complete relief from his pain. This illustrates how important it can be to desensitize the affected area, especially when deep, invasive surgery is involved.

TREATMENT OPTIONS

Self-massage

It's important to let scars heal properly, but it's also a good idea to make sure they don't harden too much. Around a month after surgery, you can use the following massage and pressure technique to help prevent scars from causing referred pain.

Massage the area of the scar with almond oil or another oil containing vitamin E. Press with your fingers around the area of the scar, and keep applying pressure until you feel tension or stiffness in this area. Maintain the pressure, and when you feel the tension and adhesions release, increase the pressure a little and wait until you feel the release again. Keep going like this for a few minutes, moving your fingers up and down and side to side. Repeat this therapy several days in a row.

Injections

I have given thousands of injections to patients, and the results can be quite remarkable. Pain in the local scarring process, which is often nervous in origin, can defy medical explanation. Sometimes, local scar pain disappears after an anesthetic is injected directly into the affected area. It doesn't necessarily stop there, though. Injections of scars following lumbar operations can noticeably reduce local pain in the lumbar region, but also have an impact on referred pain, and specifically sciatica-type pain. Isn't this intriguing? The body is full of mysteries, and it's up to us to shed light on them.

PREVENTIVE MEASURES

It's important to avoid exposing a scar to the sun for the first few weeks after an operation. Massage with vitamin E and almond oil as described above, twice a day for several weeks.

Because you're trying to rebuild the various layers of muscle, it's a good idea to boost your protein intake. Vitamin C is important, too, because it helps to build collagen.

Cut down on sugar, as well—I can never stress this enough! It's well established that scars take a long time to heal in diabetics, as well as in people who may be suffering from insulin resistance even though they haven't been diagnosed with diabetes.

Avoid cortisone creams, since they can slow the healing process and thin the skin. However, if you have thick, keloid scars, a cortisone cream can help to prevent the scars from becoming raised.

A therapist specializing in massage, osteopathy, or physiotherapy can work proactively to minimize adhesions.

Fibromyalgia

Fibromyalgia is a painful subject—not only for suffering patients but also for doctors at a loss for treatments to suggest. And that's not to mention the debate about whether or not the condition really exists. Is it a disease, and can it really be debilitating? Or is it all in the mind, as some critics maintain? In the 1970s, given its predominant incidence in women, fibromyalgia used to be considered a type of "female hysteria," alongside other psychiatric illnesses that would now be classified as depression.

I remember helping fibromyalgic patients thirty years ago and obtaining interesting results using the best of my knowledge at that time. I had gone to a seminar on the subject at the hospital where I was working; I recall being taken aback when the speaker, a female physician, described the disease as a psychiatric disorder and explained that patients simply needed to pull themselves together! Unfortunately, this kind of skepticism is still common among many doctors. When the medical establishment has no pharmaceutical solution for a condition and no scientific, physical explanation for its origin, it's inclined to discredit the condition and label it a "psychological disorder." Let's shed some light on this somewhat poorly defined condition that afflicts too many people.

RECOGNITION FOR THE DISEASE TODAY

Fibromyalgia stems from "fibro" (meaning fibrous or fibrosis) and "myalgia" (meaning muscle pain). It's used to define a condition similar to muscular rheumatism, in that the muscles are hypersensitive. This isn't a new concept. As early as the 1900s, some doctors were talking about "fibrositis" or "fibromyositis." Long rejected as a physical disease by physicians—as described above, it used to be considered a psychological disorder—fibromyalgia was finally recognized by the World Health Organization as a rheumatic disease in 1992. Then, in the early 2000s, scientific breakthroughs proved that the neuromuscular aspect was tied to deficiencies of the neurotransmitters dopamine, serotonin, and noradrenalin.[3] More recently, several researchers, together with the Institute for Functional Medicine in the United States, have focused on the condition as an issue related to a dysfunction in the intracellular mitochondria (small particles in the cells that deliver energy throughout the body, to the brain as well as the muscles).[4] Since the advent of MRIS, we've been able to see anomalies in patients with fibromyalgia in parts of the brain correlated with pain.[5] Fibromyalgia is therefore a phenomenon with physical and physiological manifestations, associated with secondary psychological effects.

While it's classified as a disease, I prefer to think of fibromyalgia as a combination of symptoms that can be hard to define. "Fibromyalgia syndrome" would be a more accurate term, as a syndrome comprises a multitude of signs and symptoms, and there are still no specific laboratory tests to detect the condition. I've always treated patients afflicted by this condition by seeking the underlying cause. And despite it being thought of as a chronic illness unlikely to find a cure, a great many of my patients have managed to rid themselves of fibromyalgia for good. You don't necessarily have to resign yourself to suffering from this condition for the rest of your life.

It's well worth exploring this topic in depth, because a significant percentage of the population is said to suffer from fibromyalgia—mainly women, and sometimes even children. Fibromyalgia affects close to a million Canadians, while in the United States estimates suggest that between four and ten million Americans are living with the condition.[6]

In the past I've struggled to get patients' insurance companies to recognize their fibromyalgia as a disability. Today, however, this condition is widely recognized and accepted as a valid reason for a disability claim, although this does often require an expert physician's opinion. A considerable percentage of sufferers find their ability to perform daily activities is significantly diminished. Some may have to stop working entirely, although this can often be avoided once we've addressed the underlying causes. In some cases, I've prepared a customized program for incapacitated patients whose insurance companies agreed to cover the costs of treatment beyond the short-term disability period. This has been a win-win solution; the patient could return to work and the insurance company avoided paying long-term disability benefits.

All in all, much of the skepticism in the medical community surrounding fibromyalgia has dissipated since the neurophysiological mechanisms of the condition have come to light. However, many patients do still report frustration at the lack of credibility they're given, with some caregivers viewing their symptoms as psychosomatic or ascribing them to hypochondria. Here it's crucial for there to be a relationship of trust between doctor and patient. If patients are treated with empathy and feel they can trust their therapist, they'll be less inclined to overmedicate and waste appointment time.

CHALLENGES IN ESTABLISHING A DIAGNOSIS

Fibromyalgia can be challenging to diagnose as the symptoms are often vague and inconsistent in the beginning. The pain is there in the muscles, but it takes at least three months, and over six months in some cases, to establish a diagnosis.

Patients usually report widespread pain, often in the upper body, sometimes in the lower body, and occasionally in both. Pain isn't necessarily confined to the muscles; sometimes the joints are also affected, despite a lack of the inflammation found in arthritis. Pressure on the muscles, stress, weather, and overly vigorous exercise can all affect the intensity of the pain.

In some cases, fibromyalgia may be connected with other conditions, such as irritable bowel syndrome, chronic fatigue, mood disorders, migraines, premenstrual syndrome, food intolerances, local and sometimes generalized myofascial pain syndrome, temporomandibular joint dysfunction (with painful jaw clicking), and even urinary symptoms including cystitis and overactive bladder.[7] This may suggest certain links between these conditions and raise questions of cause and effect. We'll explore this shortly, because it's important to treat the cause and not just the symptoms.

Fibromyalgia points

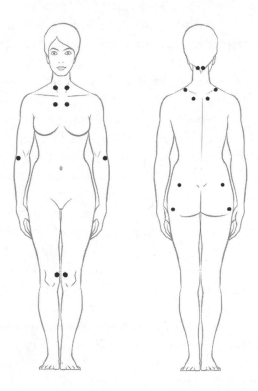

Traditionally, at least eleven of these eighteen fibromyalgia points—determined by the American College of Rheumatology in 1990 and found in most patients—must be present to establish a fibromyalgia (FM) diagnosis. Under the Canadian National Guidelines, we're increasingly moving away from these eighteen tender points and considering a patient's broader symptoms instead, since muscle pain has been seen to manifest elsewhere too. Often, there are just a few painful areas in the beginning, and a spread is observed over time. As a result, it's important to bear in mind that a diagnosis may only be confirmed after several appointments and on the basis of the overall symptoms.

What kinds of tests can patients with this type of pain syndrome undergo? Unfortunately, lab tests are of little use in establishing an FM diagnosis, and embarking on a long investigation can be not only fruitless but also detrimental to the patient's well-being. Basic screening involves a complete blood analysis (including sedimentation, C-reactive protein, thyroid screen, and creatine kinase) and clinical assessment to rule out any other arthritic or neurological conditions.

Once all other conditions have been ruled out, it's important to trace the underlying causes of the fibromyalgia symptoms. Patients are typically asked to complete an in-depth questionnaire designed to detect any allergies, immunological dysfunctions, intestinal microbiota imbalance, insulin resistance, or prediabetes. That being said, in order to avoid falling into the trap of never-ending tests, making the patient feel increasingly insecure, doctors must seek to establish an FM diagnosis as early as possible, unless new signs or symptoms point toward other conditions (such as arthritis, connective tissue diseases, neurological diseases such as multiple sclerosis, or neuromuscular diseases). Hypothyroidism should be explored as a possibility right from the outset, as it can cause considerable fatigue and even symptoms of depression. Family doctors are generally more than able to treat fibromyalgic patients and may refer them to a relevant specialist if another condition seems to be involved.

When patients receive a fibromyalgia diagnosis, it's important for them to try to maintain a positive outlook, to avoid spiraling into depression by imagining themselves losing all enjoyment in life or becoming completely immobile. Unfortunately, because fibromyalgia is often considered a degenerative chronic condition that precludes any return to health, I've seen too many patients who lost hope when they were given a pessimistic diagnosis. Obviously, there's no miracle drug that will cure fibromyalgia—hence the importance of swimming upstream in search of a possible cause.

MULTIPLE CAUSES CAN MUDDY THE WATERS

The causes of fibromyalgia are poorly understood, because there is no single cause; this syndrome has many causal factors and manifestations depending on individual patients and their predispositions. As such, there is no universal treatment; therapy is typically tailored to the individual, taking into account the factors thought to have prompted the condition. This is why such an in-depth questionnaire is required, to figure out what may have happened in the past to trigger the onset.

Sometimes fibromyalgia can develop following a viral infection that sets the whole body off balance, generating fatigue and muscle pain. Special care should be taken with patients who are on statins, which are prescribed for life—often in high doses—and cause damage to muscle cells, leading to muscle pain and fatigue. Some breast cancer drugs, such as Femara and Arimidex, as well as bisphosphonates, used to treat osteoporosis, can also have similar effects.

According to one theory, fibromyalgia is a neurohormonal imbalance that causes hypersensitivity of the central nervous system. Think about how painful and sensitive a muscle can be after exercise—now imagine this hypersensitivity being amplified in the brain, causing extreme intensity of the pain. In fibromyalgia patients, various abnormal neurological circuits have been observed in the central nervous system and autonomic (sympathetic) nervous system, leading to heightened pain perception.[8]

As mentioned earlier, current research suggests that these patients may have a type of disorder in the mitochondria, which deliver the energy cells need to do their job. Therefore it's hardly surprising that these individuals would be experiencing fatigue and pain. Fibromyalgia is essentially an energy problem. One of the ways the body produces energy is by **glycolysis**—in other words, by breaking down sugar. However, this is an inefficient process that also produces a lot of lactic acid. It's commonly known that athletes who train too hard and for too long will produce a lot of lactic acid, which will lead to pain. Fibromyalgia patients are no strangers to the fact that a muscle that contains lactic acid hurts. Athletes can deal with this problem simply by reducing the intensity of their exercise; they will quickly get rid of the lactic acid and restore oxygen to the muscle. However, this doesn't work for people with fibromyalgia.[9] A significant buildup of lactic acid will cause them fatigue and pain and eventually lead to microtears in the muscles (including the heart, which we can't forget is a muscle too). Fibromyalgia sufferers have no recovery mechanism, and the process to eliminate toxins and repair the body functions too slowly.

Heavy-metal poisoning has been cited as another possible cause. Some patients have had dental work done with mercury and lead, which are thought to modulate brain cell sensitivity. More information about mercury and lead can be found in Chapter 5.

A genetic predisposition to fibromyalgia has been cited in some 25 percent of cases, but no defective genes per se have been identified to date. Genetic polymorphism is suspected to be to blame: in other words, the morphological nature of the otherwise normal genes in some individuals with fibromyalgia may manifest differently. The chemical compounds released by the brain (neurotransmitters) may therefore cause individuals with fibromyalgia to feel pain differently, at a greater intensity than normal, as if the neurotransmitters were amplifying the pain signals sent to the brain.

Psychological distress may hasten the onset of fibromyalgia. The stress of any physical, psychological, or sexual abuse early in life predisposes adults to health vulnerability and can be a trigger factor for fibromyalgia.[10]

Jenny was a patient who consulted me for widespread pain and fatigue that she had been experiencing for the last year or so. After doing a questionnaire, a thorough examination, and several lab tests to rule out some other serious illnesses, it became clear that hers was a case of progressive fibromyalgia associated with depression. This was consistent with the diagnosis she had been given by another doctor and for which she was taking antidepressants and painkillers. However, Jenny wanted to get to the bottom of what was wrong with her and stop taking her medication, which wasn't doing much good, in her estimation. She still felt very tired, to such an extent that she was unable to work.

I knew this patient quite well, having been her doctor for around ten years, though her last visit to me dated back five years or so. Back then, Jenny was a bubbly person who enjoyed life to the fullest. She had always been in excellent health, she exercised regularly, and thanks to her cheerful personality she had a good circle of friends. She had no children and seemed happy with the man she had been sharing her life with for the last five years.

I noticed this time that she had changed a lot physically. She told me that she had gained more than forty-five pounds over the past two years and that her relationship had gone through so many ups and downs that she and her partner had separated the previous year. Such upheavals naturally have some consequences. But what could have happened that was so bad she had gained so much weight, gone through a separation, spiraled into depression, and developed this fibromyalgia syndrome?

When I had last seen her, five years earlier, Jenny had told me that as a teenager she had had an incestuous relationship with her father, which had lasted until she turned eighteen. She told me that she loved and respected her father, that they were still on good terms, and that at the time she had even enjoyed the relationship, but that she had simply decided to put an end to a situation that would have been embarrassing if anyone had found out about it. She viewed their relationship as an expression of their affection, even though she could see how other people might find it immoral. She didn't appear to be suffering from what had happened all those years ago and described it as a thing of the past.

Now, five years later, depression and apathy were written all over her face. I could sense that she was holding something back. She could barely look at me and her eyes were scanning the floor as if she were trying to find the right words to say. Then, suddenly, she burst into tears.

Unable to contain the guilt and shame any longer, Jenny told me how her perception of the incestuous relationship with her father had changed;

how she felt she had made a grave mistake and had taken part in a crime for which she could never forgive herself. I looked at her with empathy and asked her how her view of those past events had changed so much.

Now she told me how over a year ago she had started to come across revelations about incest in the newspapers, on the radio, and on television. She had heard the stories of some remarkable people who had experienced incest or been sexually abused at an early age and now, as adults, felt outraged about it. Many people's lives had been broken by these events, and they were now exposing what had happened. Some of the perpetrators were reported to the police and given long jail sentences.

Suddenly, Jenny was struck by the full force of what had happened to her. Now she could see her father's actions as depraved offenses that were punishable by imprisonment. She still loved her father, though, and couldn't imagine him behind bars. Since this realization, she had cut off all contact with him. She felt terribly guilty and now had mixed feelings toward him. She felt pathetic, shattered; she was suffering in her entire being, her every muscle battered and bruised. All the joy had gone from her life.

As this had only happened a year or so ago, it was relatively easy for me to make the connection and explain that her physical and psychological condition could be largely a product of her coming to terms with her teenage experience.

In the year that followed, Jenny made peace with herself and managed to reach a place of complete forgiveness. She then talked to her father and explained what she had come to understand. Thanks to making the right lifestyle choices, having adequate psychotherapy, and starting to exercise again, Jenny found her pain gradually fading away, and she has now regained her zest for life.

TREATMENT OPTIONS

As we've seen, there's no miracle drug to cure fibromyalgia. It's important to treat the causes of the syndrome; as these are multiple, any treatment must be personalized, with every angle approached at the same time and in a complementary way. The following medications, however, may be helpful in relieving fibromyalgia symptoms:

- Pregabalin (Lyrica) and gabapentin (Neurontin), two antiepileptics with analgesic properties, are used to control pain in fibromyalgic patients, but the side effects can be problematic.

- One antidepressant, duloxetine (Cymbalta), can relieve symptoms of pain and depression, but research has often discredited this drug due to its undesirable side effects. Other antidepressants, such as amitriptyline (Elavil) can improve sleep and alleviate the pain.

- Anti-inflammatories such as ibuprofen (Motrin, Advil) can be used during acute phases, while painkillers such as acetaminophen (Tylenol) or tramadol can provide relief.

- And, especially as it's such a timely topic, let's not forget cannabis. In recent years, I have been using cannabis—more specifically, cannabidiol (CBD), one of the chemical compounds found in the cannabis plant—to treat individuals with fibromyalgia, as I have found that it has helped many patients who are suffering. CBD is certainly one of the most inoffensive substances used to treat chronic fibromyalgia pain. CBD is an effective painkiller and anti-inflammatory, but it is not addictive and it does not have a euphoric effect (in other words, it will not make you "high"). This treatment is well worth trying, but it should not be seen as a miracle solution, because some patients may find it does not bring them the relief they were hoping for. To increase the pain-relieving effect, sufferers may wish to add a small amount of THC (tetrahydrocannabinol, the chemical compound in cannabis that produces a psychoactive effect). To learn more about cannabis and pain relief, see Chapter 5.

- Some studies have shown clinical interest for naltrexone (Nalorex), which is typically used to reverse the effects of opioids when treating alcohol and opiate addiction. Some fibromyalgia patients seem to have responded favorably to this drug in in very low doses (3–5 mg).

Ultimately, as we've already said, treatment must target the source of the fibromyalgia. To do so, it's important to consider the immune-brain loop that triggered the syndrome and look at physiological disruptions creating lactic acid in the body and a loss of mitochondrial function. The following treatments and approaches may be helpful:

- To function properly, the mitochondria need vitamin B3, magnesium, D-ribose (a simple sugar present in all cells, required by the body to produce energy), coenzyme Q10 (CoQ10), and acetyl-L-carnitine (an amino acid), all of which can help to reduce lactic acid levels.

- Often there will be an antioxidant or hormone (principally thyroid) imbalance to correct. A diet low in sugar that will not create a rebound insulin effect—which leads to more inflammation—may be prescribed.

- Moderate exercise will drain the muscles and promote oxygen delivery. *Moderate* is the key word here, because we all know how difficult it can be to exercise when we're tired and suffering. Besides, as a general rule, if we do too much exercise, our bodies will produce more lactic acid, which is the source of the pain for those with fibromyalgia. Most people find during exercise that any muscle pain will quickly dissipate after a short rest and a few deep breaths, and they can continue their workout. That's not the case for fibromyalgia sufferers, however. Their muscles get stuck in the lactic phase and keep releasing excess oxidative free radicals; this stage can last for several hours or even days. This is where vitamin B12 can be useful for flushing free radicals out of the muscles.

- It's important to check for a potential disruption of the intestinal microbiota and supplement accordingly if need be. A good place to start is by using the 5Rs method (see Chapter 4), and first removing what is toxic, on both a physical and psychological level. This involves avoiding or limiting all elements that may be harmful, especially for those who are hypersensitive, such as mercury, aluminum, tobacco, certain drugs including statins, and air pollution. Then the right nutrients can be reintroduced to repair the gastrointestinal system.

- Overall nutrition should also be considered. Plenty has been written about the connection between nutrition and health, and some correlations have been established between fibromyalgia and gluten intolerance.

- In terms of supplements, magnesium in 300–400 mg doses, as well as potassium, can relieve muscle tension. Malic acid, which is found in most produce, including apples, pears, and grapes, can also bring improvement.

- Given the preponderance of fatigue and negative feelings in patients with fibromyalgia, likely due to neurotransmitter anomalies, supplements that promote serotonin, such as St. John's wort and 5-HTP, can help with sleep and depression. Let's not forget omega-3s, either, which stimulate brain function and reduce inflammation.

- Managing stress can not only reduce pain but also relieve symptoms of anxiety and depression.

- Psychotherapy is sometimes the key to unlocking any unresolved emotional challenges that may have triggered fibromyalgia. This condition may in fact be linked to an overflow of mismanaged emotions that end up affecting the body. Even if the physical symptoms may have their root in emotional issues, though, that doesn't make the disease or its symptoms less real.

- Acupuncture has proven to be effective at reducing pain and depression and promoting sleep in fibromyalgia patients.[11]

- Massage can also help, provided that it's done gently, because a vigorous massage can exacerbate the pain.

- Injecting the trigger points with a low-dilution cortisone solution combined with a painkiller, such as xylocaine or procaine, may help to reduce muscle pain (see Chapter 6). In Europe and the United States, very low dilutions of procaine anesthetics are combined with various natural substances, including endorphins, collagen, antioxidants, growth factors, and anti-inflammatories such as interleukins, to relieve pain, reduce local inflammation, and promote tissue regeneration. Hopes are high for these safe injection techniques and their highly promising results. The same techniques are also used to treat myofascial and joint conditions.

Headaches

Headaches are a regular pain in the lives of many thousands of people. Most of the time headaches aren't serious, but they're still a major reason for seeking medical advice.

The term *headache* covers a multitude of conditions, including tension headaches, migraines, sinusitis, occipital neuralgia, and cluster headaches.

TENSION HEADACHES

Without a doubt, these are the most frequent type of headaches. While they're not dangerous, they can still severely disrupt our quality of life. Most of us will experience this type of headache at some point in our lives, often following times of psychological stress or effort, such as spending a long time at a computer, which can generate muscle tension in the neck and shoulders and bring on a headache. This type of headache causes a stabbing pain that tends to get worse at the end of the day. It's generally felt on both sides of the head and has been likened to wearing a hat that's too small.

MIGRAINES

Let's talk about the notorious head pain we call migraine. The term is often misused to refer to a wide range of head pains, but a true migraine is much more intense and complex than other types of headaches and can even lead to nervous system disorders.

A true migraine is characterized by a headache that lasts between four and seventy-two hours, with a throbbing pain that's generally located on one side of the head—sometimes the left, sometimes the right. Rapid movement usually worsens the pain. Migraines are frequently accompanied by nausea, vomiting, or sensitivity to light or sound. Interestingly, migraines are not caused by a wound or damage to an organ; even if the symptoms can seem concerning, there will be no aftereffects on the brain or vision.

Migraine sufferers frequently report experiencing symptoms known as a *prodrome* or *aura* before the pain sets in. These symptoms, which typically last around half an hour, may include yawning, mood changes, blurred vision, seeing flickering lights, or sometimes numbness in a limb. Rest assured, this has nothing to do with a stroke (cerebrovascular accident) or hypertensive crisis.

The tendency to get migraines is hereditary. The condition manifests differently in children, since they may rarely experience headaches. Instead, children with migraines may experience episodes of vomiting, stomachache, and motion sickness and will seem pale and fatigued.

As soon as the first warning signs of migraine appear, it's important to seek medical advice to make sure the symptoms are not secondary headaches related to a tumor, for instance, or to malignant hypertension or any other form of intercranial hypertension.

MIGRAINE CAUSES

Stress and overwork play a significant role in the occurrence of migraines. Women are also more likely to get migraines when they are menstruating.

According to some experts, certain foods can trigger migraines, the most common being chocolate, dairy products (especially blue cheese), eggs, sugar, gluten, and sometimes wine and coffee. However, I've often found that coffee can defuse a migraine in its early stages.

TREATMENT OPTIONS

Among the most-prescribed drugs for migraine are propranolol (Inderal)—a drug that was formerly prescribed to treat hypertension—as well as anticonvulsants such as gabapentin (Neurontin) and antidepressants.

The use of oral anti-inflammatories such as ibuprofen (Motrin, Advil) and aspirin, or even analgesics such as acetaminophen (Tylenol) can thwart a migraine attack if taken as soon as the first signs appear. Some sufferers find that taking both of these types of drugs together works best. As soon as a migraine starts, lying down in a dark, quiet room, massaging your head and neck, and applying cold compresses to your face can ease the symptoms or even make them go away.

Triptans (Imitrex, Maxalt, Zomig) are another family of prescription drugs, introduced over fifteen years ago. They work by **serotonergic** action, constricting the blood vessels to reduce sensations of pressure in the head. These are available in tablet form, as a nasal spray, and even as a self-administered injection. Here, too, it's important to act fast as soon as prodrome or migraine symptoms appear. The earlier the treatment begins, the quicker and easier the migraine will disappear. The use of opiate drugs is not advisable. They may be more powerful painkillers, but there's a risk of addiction, drowsiness, constipation, and other side effects.

Various supplements can reduce the symptoms of a migraine or avoid triggering an attack in some sufferers. Around 60 percent of women reported experiencing a reduction in pain by taking a 400 mg vitamin B12 supplement daily. Studies have also suggested that magnesium can be beneficial for migraines. The daily recommended dose is 300–400 mg per day. One well-known antioxidant, CoQ10, has also proven effective against migraine in some 60 percent of patients at a dose of 150–200 mg daily.[12]

Another potential treatment for women of childbearing age whose hormonal fluctuations may cause or precipitate migraines is hormone replacement therapy. In my experience, the same also goes for menopausal women.

BOTOX FOR HEADACHES?

Some patients ask me about Botox injections as a cure for their headaches. Let's be clear: Botox is a bacterial toxin. Botulinum toxin is secreted by the bacterium that causes botulism, a foodborne infection contracted by consuming infected canned goods. This powerful poison attacks the motor nerves and can cause muscle paralysis. It reduces spasticity, hence its popularity in cosmetic medicine and pain treatment, as it promotes the release of muscle contractions and wrinkles.

Botox was approved by the U.S. Food and Drug Administration in 2010 for the treatment of chronic migraines. Personally, I rarely recommend this treatment, since the preventive effect of Botox is no greater than that of a placebo. Studies of nearly 1,400 patients have even shown a placebo to be slightly more effective.

What's more, Botox must be injected regularly, every three to six months, and its temporary side effects include fever, facial muscle weakness, droopy eyelids, skin rash, flu-like symptoms, breathing difficulties, and difficulty swallowing.

MIGRAINE PREVENTION

Healthy lifestyle choices, including exercise and an appropriate diet, can help to prevent migraines. As we saw earlier, some foods may increase the risk of migraine. Therefore it may be wise, depending on your tolerance, to avoid chocolate, alcohol (particularly white wine), and some cheeses, as well as too much coffee. Beware of cutting down on caffeine too suddenly, however, as this may create withdrawal symptoms and provoke headaches. If you're going to cut out coffee, it's best to reduce your consumption gradually. Coffee isn't harmful in itself, at least no more than alcohol in my estimation, but everything is always better in moderation.

One food additive that can trigger migraines is the flavor enhancer monosodium glutamate (MSG), commonly added to Chinese cuisine and to many restaurant and processed foods. In my opinion, it's far too widely and often too liberally used. If you want to avoid this additive, you'll need to learn how to decipher food labels, because it can be found lurking everywhere. Some hidden names for MSG include hydrolyzed vegetable protein, autolyzed yeast extract, soy extract, protein isolate, and E620, to name but a few. Glutamate is one of our neurotransmitters and that ingesting it through our food on a day-to-day basis can be harmful for hypersensitive individuals, as well as for anyone if consumed in too great a quantity or over too long a time. Some experiments on mice that involved ingesting large quantities of glutamate showed a correlation between this substance and the incidence of brain damage.[13] According to the Mayo Clinic, its side effects can include headache, sweating, weight gain (indirectly, because MSG stimulates appetite), a throbbing feeling in the head and temples, asthma, nausea, and weakness—to the extent that I have observed some patients slip toward unconsciousness. The debate still rages on as to the harmfulness or harmlessness of MSG. However, it seems that its harmful effects are more marked in children, as their brains are more permeable than adults' (their blood-brain barrier is more sensitive). Why not simply remove MSG from our food to eliminate the risk one day of finding out its adverse health effects the hard way? In any case, we could all probably stand to eat fewer processed foods.

OCCIPITAL NEURALGIA

Occipital neuralgia is a type of headache that usually affects one side of the head, but sometimes both. Technically speaking, it's a peripheral neuropathy in the neck that travels up to the head, and it's more common that you might think. The pain travels along the greater C2 occipital nerve—also called Arnold's nerve—hence the condition sometimes being referred to as C2 neuralgia or Arnold's neuralgia. The pain can be very intense and affects the neck, the top of the head, and even the eye. It can feel like pressure, a burning sensation, or even an electric shock. Symptoms may last from a few days to several weeks, and can even persist for years if the cause is not found.

Jasmine was a patient who came to my clinic to consult for the cranial pain she had been suffering for more than two years. She had tried all kinds of pain medication and anti-inflammatories, to no great effect. Every single day she had a headache that was often unbearably intense. She had been told she was suffering from atypical migraines. The pain was mainly in the upper right side of her head, with some pain in her forehead that often radiated behind her right eye. She presented no neurological symptoms or vision problems. She felt discomfort in her right eyebrow when I pinched and rolled this area, and winced when I applied pressure to the emergence of the second occipital nerve. It was clear to me that Jasmine was suffering from occipital neuralgia.

I told her where her pain was coming from and suggested a local injection of a xylocaine and cortisone solution to the right occipital. Two minutes later, she gave me a strange look and asked me whether it was possible for the pain to have disappeared already. I told her yes, since xylocaine acts rapidly as a local anesthetic, and thanks to the medication I used to make the injection more comfortable, that was a sure sign that we had administered the injection to the right place. She blinked and told me she felt as if she could see more clearly and her eye was more relaxed. That observation was perfectly logical, and many of my patients have had the same experience. I prescribed her some exercises for her neck similar to those described in Chapter 5. When she checked in with me a month later, she was happy to report that she no longer had to take painkillers every day and that her life was back to normal.

MYOFASCIAL PAIN SYNDROME (MPS)

Another frequent type of headache, characterized by tension in the masseter and temporal muscles we use for chewing, falls under the label of myofascial pain syndrome (MPS). Head pain may also be referred from the trapezius muscles and the muscles that attach to the shoulder blade, such as the levator scapulae muscle.

TREATMENT OPTIONS

MPS is very common, and various neck muscles and fascia can cause pain in different parts of the head. To alleviate the pain, we first need to pinpoint the muscles experiencing the abnormal tension, contractures, and knots that are causing the local or referred pain. Massaging these muscles can then help to gradually make the headaches go away. Acupuncture can also work wonders.

Injecting xylocaine locally—directly into the muscle knots using Dr. Janet Travell's technique (page 131)—will often bring complete relief. If the pain has persisted for months or years, the treatment will need to involve a series of injections to the myofascial trigger points. Because muscle tension due to anxiety and overwork is often the source of the problem, supplements such as magnesium, valerian, passionflower, and theanine can be useful in restoring muscle quality.

CLUSTER HEADACHES

Far less common than other types of headaches, cluster headaches are a series of severe recurring headaches that can last for days or weeks at a time. Symptoms tend to be focused on one side of the face and often include a red, teary, or droopy eye and a runny nose, sometimes facial swelling and sweating, and even droopy eyelids.

Attacks may occur every day, and some patients may experience up to eight in the same day. Unlike migraines, cluster headaches go away and come back again later. Attacks occur suddenly and sporadically throughout the day, and sufferers often report feeling as if their eye is going to pop out of its socket. Cluster headaches aren't aggravated by daily activities; on the contrary, patients often prefer to move around and have difficulty staying still. Cluster headache episodes are followed by long periods of no pain. The causes of the condition are still unclear, but factors such as alcohol and stress are thought to be involved.

TREATMENT OPTIONS

Treatment is more complex for cluster headaches than for other types of headaches, and medical advice should be sought both for prevention and for the acute phase of the condition.

Neck pain

Neck pain is the reason for more than ten million medical appointments a year in the United States.[14] Around half of all Americans experience it every year. Neck pain (or cervicodynia) can extend from the back of the head (occiput) down to the shoulder blades. We don't always realize it, but pain between the shoulder blades—interscapular pain, to be precise—often stems from a pain in the neck.[15] The injury is local, but the pain can also be felt remotely.

The pain can sometimes hinder movement in the neck, particularly rotation, flexion, and extension. It may radiate to the upper limbs and travel down the nerves to the upper arms, forearms, and hands. It's not uncommon for sufferers to feel numbness in the upper limbs. The term for this is paresthesia of the extremities, and the source may well lie in the neck area. Remember that neck pain is a symptom rather than a diagnosis. That's why it's important to identify the cause of the pain and the source of the injury.

Neck pain can develop over time. The most common cause today is physical tension brought on by the stationary postures of computer-based work. When we spend long hours in front of a screen, there is constant muscle tension in our neck and shoulders.

CERVICAL DISC INJURY

Neck pain may be caused by a cervical disc injury attributable to either chronic degeneration or acute trauma (a shock or blow to the neck). Generally with a disc injury, the patient will feel pain radiating down the nerve to the left or right shoulder as well as the pain in the neck. There may also be some numbness or tingling.

This area may also be the source of a herniated disc (see page 236). This term refers to a protrusion (swelling) of the gel-like disc center that leaks to the outside of the disc through tears in the fibers. This causes part of the disc to spill into the spinal canal, which can compress the emergence of a cervical nerve, causing pain, numbness, and ultimately deterioration of the motor nerve—and a loss of strength in one of the upper limbs.

The majority of cases do not call for surgery. Even if radiographs show a disc injury, the symptoms will be the determining factors. If the patient feels pinching, numbness and tingling, and a loss of strength in the upper limbs, a conservative medical treatment approach will first be taken, using NSAIDs (typically ibuprofen or aspirin), other analgesics, muscle relaxants, physical rehabilitation, and sometimes injections.

If medical treatment fails, surgical intervention may be considered.

CERVICAL OSTEOARTHRITIS

One frequent manifestation of neck pain in seniors is cervical osteoarthritis, which can also cause headaches. Don't be too quick to blame osteoarthritis for neck pain, though. While it can cause pain along the spine, it's not as widespread as you might think. Many people's X-rays show a remarkable degree of osteoarthritis, yet they never feel any neck, back, or lumbar pain there aren't necessarily parallels between the severity of osteoarthritis and the symptoms experienced by the person. It's the doctor's job to find the exact correlation between the symptoms described by the patient and the findings from the radiograph. As I often say, we don't treat the X-ray, we treat the patient!

SPASMODIC TORTICOLLIS

Spasmodic torticollis (or cervical dystonia) is a painful condition whereby the muscles on one side of the neck contract involuntarily and cause the head to lean to the side. This position is not only impossible to control, it's uncomfortable and can be very bothersome.

The symptoms will typically disappear just as gradually as they appear. While there is no treatment to relieve the tension per se, Botox (botulinum toxin) injections can help to relax the muscles and alleviate the symptoms. These injections can be therapeutically effective for several months, which is usually long enough for things to clear up.

Neck trauma (whiplash)

Whiplash is a term that refers to the sudden and sharp forward-and-backward movement of the head and neck that can occur in a car crash. After a trauma like this, it's not uncommon for patients to experience dizziness and feel like they're losing their balance, as well as feeling pain in the back of their head and toward the front of their head around their eyes. These headaches, unlike migraines, may persist for days, weeks, or months. Until the source of the problem is identified, patients may take medication to relieve the headaches, but without lasting results.

Whiplash is really just a sprained neck. It occurs during rapid deceleration, and injuries can be significant even in low-speed impacts. After a fender bender we can often be amazed at how little damage there seems to be to the car, without realizing that we're the ones who've suffered the most damage! In whiplash, the neck undergoes rapid flexion followed by hyperextension. It's this back-and-forth movement of the head that can create immense tension in the cervical spine. This tension can affect many of the small ligaments holding the vertebrae together, causing stretching and even microtears. The shock can sometimes even cause disc injuries, as well as putting the entire muscle mass and tendons of the neck under violent stress. The pain can be very intense, to the point of causing a loss of mobility. Sometimes, simply supporting the weight of the head in a standing position can be difficult. Rotating the head can also be painful and limited.

Besides dizziness, patients may experience fatigue and have trouble concentrating. In most cases, nothing will show up on X-rays, scans, or MRIs. While radiology may have a hard time detecting whiplash as such, a deviation from the normal curve of the neck may be observed. Complementary MRI exams may be ordered if there are neurological symptoms, such as numbness or weakness in the upper limbs.

PREVENTION OF WHIPLASH (AND HEAD INJURIES)

By definition, car accidents are hard to avoid, but the least you can do is to ensure that the headrest of your seat is positioned so that it prevents the head from snapping backward in the event of an impact. Steering-wheel and side-curtain airbags will also greatly help to reduce potential injury to the head and neck.

Beware of extreme or action sports that involve rapid, jerking movements of the head—these are essentially mini-whiplashes![16] The same goes for any sports that may cause bruising to the head and neck, which can cause neck pain, headaches, poor balance, or even mood disorders that may lead to depression. Evidence has shown that some boxers who have suffered multiple concussions have ended up developing psychological disorders, with several even committing suicide.[17] Indeed, all contact sports involving repeated hits to the head can lead to lasting side effects, though some of them—such as mood and sleep disorders, trouble concentrating, coordination issues, learning difficulties, impatience, and aggression—may not always be linked back to the head injuries. All of these side effects can affect a patient's personality and social skills, however, and can even lead to unexplained withdrawal behavior.

Caution is the name of the game when it comes to protecting this crucial organ of ours! Despite being protected by the bony structure of the skull, the brain is still a spongy mass that can be significantly compressed under impact. Tiny blood vessels can burst, edemas can form, and even the nerve structure can be altered. Concussions are not without consequence, and even if the individual seems to have recovered physically, it's not uncommon for fatigue and memory and concentration issues to persist for months or years. I can't help but caution against riding extreme roller coasters, too. Although there are no impacts to speak of, the sudden acceleration and deceleration can be enough to cause neck and head injuries.[18]

Scoliosis

Scoliosis is a condition featuring an abnormal S-shaped curvature of the spine. (Lordosis, another disorder that is similarly characterized by an exaggerated curve to the spine, is rarely painful.) The most frequent cause of scoliosis is poor posture, particularly in individuals who spend long hours working in a seated position. In fact, seated work can lead not only to scoliosis, but also to hip problems.

Some forms of scoliosis are caused by having one leg shorter than the other, for example in individuals who have suffered from polio— in which case, the polio compensates for the asymmetry. Scoliosis in other individuals may be caused by a pelvic rotation disorder. The spine rests on the sacrum, and if the pelvis is rotated or off balance, the spine starts from an asymmetrical foundation and has to correct its upward trajectory. To ensure the head is centered, the spine may curve first to the left, for example, then to the right until it's straight.

TREATMENT OPTIONS

Scoliosis doesn't necessarily require surgery, unless it is highly pronounced. If diagnosed after adolescence, the curvature will remain, as the spine stops growing at some point during the teenage years. In cases of mild scoliosis, it can be preferable to target the cause, which may lie in the pelvis or the feet, and correct it with appropriate exercises and foot orthotics.

For example, scoliosis caused by flat feet can be treated with corrective orthotics that support the arch of the foot. Some posturologists and osteopaths take a different approach to this problem. If the tension stemming from the feet is not symmetrical, the entire muscle and tendon load of the knee and hip will twist the spine. In many cases, a progressive therapy with certain exercises and special soles can apply precise pressure to the plantar arch with a view to correcting the situation. This approach uses the patient's own muscle mass to gradually realign the spine.

While not everyone agrees with this theory, the results are sometimes astounding. This approach tends to be widespread in France, whereas the traditional North American approach tends to correct the effect of the scoliosis rather than the cause. Here, if the foot is flat, we correct the arch, and if one leg is shorter than the other, we modify the heel of the shoe on the shorter leg to even things out.

Scoliosis pain develops over the long term. In young people, who are often very active and play lots of sports, the spine tends to do well, but by their fifties, back pain may manifest as a result of the scoliosis, which will have ingrained certain issues over time.

Many cases of scoliosis can be treated by proper realignment of the spine through osteopathy, wearing proper orthotics, and working with the feet, legs, and hips to restore a natural curve to the spine.[19] Problematic cases of scoliosis will require radiological assessment and should be treated by a specialist.

Herniated discs

The classic case of a herniated lumbar disc—or slipped disc—happens when part of the disc swells and protrudes, compressing the sciatic nerve. Patients present with low back pain that radiates into the leg, making it excruciatingly painful for them to move around.

Today, thanks to MRIs, we can clearly see the intervertebral discs and detect an array of conditions ranging from mild disc swelling to severe herniated discs. Doctors must avoid falling into the trap of interpreting a protrusion, bulging, or mild herniated disc as the cause of back or sciatic pain. Over time, the discs will wear and dry out, and may sometimes crack, but they aren't necessarily a source of pain as such. Did you know that 15 percent of herniated discs detected by MRIs are found in patients with no symptoms at all?[20] As well as using medical imaging, doctors must also perform a proper palpatory examination. In other words, they have to actually touch their patient!

The vast majority of herniated discs diagnosed radiologically and clinically may clear up on their own over time. How exactly can a disc herniation resorb, or repair itself, on its own? Basically, the body will try to repair itself. If the protuberance in the disc is far from the nerve, often there will be no neurological issues, so no operation will be necessary. If the disc is pressing lightly on the nerve, the disc will tend to turn in on itself a little as the inflammation subsides, and this is often enough for the symptoms to disappear, even though an X-ray may still show a herniated disc. As the swelling in the disc goes down (inflammation assumes the tissues will expand), the herniation resorbs itself.

TREATMENT OPTIONS

Rest and heat

We're often told that it's important to keep moving and not stay still when we have back pain. This is true for chronic back pain. However, during the acute phase, it's crucial to rest and limit movement to give the inflammation time to subside and allow the body to recover.

Physiotherapy

Physiotherapy can improve the condition and promote a faster return to health. When the symptoms have calmed down and the patient feels more mobile, the doctor may prescribe physical rehabilitation exercises to improve posture, flexibility, and core and back strength.

Injections

A local injection of cortisone-based anti-inflammatories and muscle relaxants or anesthetics can accelerate the spontaneous resorption mentioned earlier. Epidural steroid injections close to the emergence of the nerve can often bring significant progress and speed up a complete recovery. I've done around a thousand caudal epidurals (at the end of the sacrum) that have been surprisingly effective, even for pain that has persisted for months or years.

Injections of enzymes such as chymopapain can also be administered directly to the disc; they work by dissolving the part of the disc that is compressing the nerve. This technique is used very little, however. One thing to bear in mind is that there are a number of substances, including fatty tissue, separating the nerve from the disc. According to the theory of homeostasis, because the body has a natural tendency to try to rebalance itself and reduce the pain, the surrounding fatty tissue may gradually resorb, leaving more space for the nerve.

Surgery

In the past, doctors used to operate regularly on patients presenting with a herniated disc, and often there would be complications or a recurrence. Over time, we came to understand that by selecting those cases most likely to benefit from surgery, the incidence of recurrence would be much lower. Today, the decision to operate on a herniated disc—a procedure called a **discectomy**—is typically made if the symptoms persist, or if there are neurological signs in the lower limbs, such as a loss of strength or numbness in the legs, muscular atrophy, or abolished reflexes (an absence of movement in the leg when the knee is tapped with a little hammer—a sign that the nerve is afflicted). Surgery is also indicated in cases of **cauda equina syndrome**. This condition manifests as a large herniated disc compressing the nerves that lead to the genital and sphincter organs, and is often considered a surgical emergency.

It's important to remember that there are risks associated with surgery, particularly the risk of local infection or damaging the nerve itself—which may cause numbness or even partial paralysis of a limb—as well as fibrous scars that can often be painful in themselves. Surgically excising a disc will also have mechanical stress impacts on the other vertebrae.

Bear in mind that only 5 to 10 percent of herniated disc cases may require surgery, and that a healthy lifestyle that includes regular exercise and correct weight-lifting technique (bend the knees rather than the back) remains the best prevention.

Epicondylitis (tennis elbow)

Epicondylitis, or tennis elbow, as it's more commonly known, is a common and painful condition that can occur even if you've never touched a tennis racket in your life. This is a form of tendinitis in the **epicondyle**, the small bony protuberance on the outside of the elbow where the muscles that extend the wrist and hand are attached. Pain is felt in the elbow itself and may radiate into the forearm and sometimes down to the hand. Often, patients will feel they have so little strength, they find it hard to even pick up a bottle from a table.

This condition tends to develop as a result of repetitive forearm movements and overexertion, but it can creep up gradually and strike without warning, even without an underlying trauma. The tendon degenerates at its insertion point for reasons that are sometimes unclear, which leads to local microtearing or a breakdown of the tendon fibers. Cervical (neck) problems can sometimes cause or be conducive to irritability in the nerve components of the elbow and its tendons, leading to pain, inflammation, and often chronic **tendinosis** (softening of the tendon).

This condition can be caused by intense effort or exercise without warming up. In fact, I've often seen patients present with this condition after reaching around from the front seat of their car to pick up a heavy bag from the back seat. The movement of stretching their extended arm out to pick up the bag exerts undue stress on the tendons in the elbow.

This type of pain can last for months but will often resolve itself over time, and so it's easy to believe that the medication taken during this time did all the healing work. However, it's important not to be lulled into a false sense of security, since taking painkillers so that you can keep doing your regular activities regardless can aggravate the situation.

TREATMENT OPTIONS

Various treatments can nip tennis elbow in the bud and help sufferers get back to normal. In 90 percent of cases, physiotherapy, chiropractic treatment, acupuncture, injections with or without corticosteroids, and deep friction massage of the elbow can resolve the issue, as can icing and massaging the epicondyle and carpal extensor muscle. In 5 to 10 percent of cases, if the condition has become chronic and various treatments have not worked, surgery may deliver lasting results.[21]

Epicondylitis (tennis elbow)

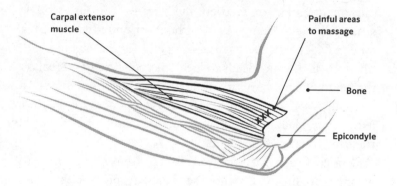

Carpal extensor muscle

Painful areas to massage

Bone

Epicondyle

Carpal tunnel syndrome

This syndrome is characterized by a compression of the median nerve at the wrist. The carpal tunnel becomes too narrow when there is inflammation in the tendons, and the median nerve ends up being compressed. This causes **paresthesias**, or numbness.

Carpal tunnel syndrome

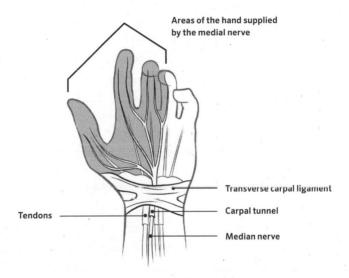

Areas of the hand supplied by the medial nerve

Transverse carpal ligament

Carpal tunnel

Tendons

Median nerve

This numbness in the hands is frequently accompanied by pain. Symptoms tend to be worse at night and sufferers can find themselves waking up and having to shake the painful pins and needles out of their hands. If the condition worsens, they may experience a loss of strength and mobility in their fingers—specifically the thumb and the first three fingers. The little finger will be unaffected as it's supplied by a different nerve.

This congestion in the carpal tunnel is often due to repeated movements, long hours spent at a computer with poor posture, or working with vibrating or hammering tools, such as a jackhammer. Sometimes, if there is osteoarthritis in the wrist or arthritis with swelling in the bones of the wrist, the nerve can also be compressed, with the same consequences. There is a risk of atrophy in the muscles of the hand if the problem persists.

This phenomenon can also occur in pregnant women or individuals with a thyroid disorder when there is a buildup of fluid (edema) in the wrist.[22] We must start by treating the cause, either by fixing the thyroid problems or changing the way we work.

TREATMENT OPTIONS

Vitamin B6 can help restore function to the nerve. Various local treatments can provide relief and promote healing—namely physiotherapy, chiropractic, and acupuncture—as well as taking NSAIDs.

A local injection or two in the wrist can deliver a quick fix, but it will take some exercises to prevent any recurrence. Sometimes, stretching exercises alone can be enough to avoid compression and keep the nerve running smoothly along the tendons. Failing that, surgery can be an alternative solution.

Below you'll find a series of five exercises to promote mobility and ensure a smooth course for the median nerve. The idea is to gently stretch the median nerve from the neck all the way down to the fingers. The key thing is to extend the wrist in various positions with the arm outstretched completely. The arrows indicate the direction of the movement. You can also see these exercises on my website at drbrouillard.com.

Exercises for carpal tunnel syndrome

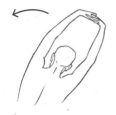

Extend one arm fully in front of you, palm facing up, and point your fingers downward. Reach for your fingers with your other hand and pull them gently toward you. Hold for five seconds. Release the pressure a little, then pull again with more pressure. Repeat ten times.

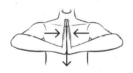

Stretch your arms overhead, interlace your fingers, and turn your palms out. Now lean your torso from side to side, pushing as hard and stretching as high as you can. Repeat ten times.

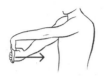

Press your palms together in front of your chest, then lower your arms as far as you can without separating your palms. Release the pressure a little and then push your palms together again a little harder. Repeat ten times.

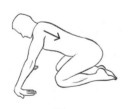

Kneel down tall and stretch your arms out in front of you with your fingers pointing toward your knees. Slowly slide your back down as if you were trying to sit on your heels. Hold for around ten seconds. You should feel increasing tension in your forearms as you bring your buttocks back toward your heels. Now lift your buttocks a little, then try to sit down toward your heels again. Repeat five times.

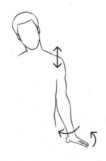

Extend one arm by your side with your fingers pointed forward and extend your wrist. Tilt your head to the opposite side, then pump your extended arm up and down from the shoulder. Continue this movement for three minutes, keeping your arm, wrist, and fingers fully extended. Repeat three times a day.

Algodystrophy

Also known as **complex regional pain syndrome**, algodystrophy is a poorly understood pathological condition characterized by various pains in the limbs as a result of a trauma, amputation, fracture, surgery, injection, or sometimes even a mild injury. I once treated a nurse who found herself suffering from this syndrome after a simple vaccination. Even if the underlying cause seems minor, it's important to see a doctor if you find yourself experiencing symptoms of algodystrophy.

The problem lies with the nerves surrounding the injury, which react erratically in a completely dysfunctional way. Often, the sympathetic nervous system reacts drastically, creating painful muscle contractions and vascular changes with edema (swelling and bloating) in the affected limb. Frequently the bone will tend to demineralize, and there will be changes in skin color and temperature.[23]

TREATMENT OPTIONS

Sometimes a small injury or wound can trigger a reaction of the sympathetic nervous system and initiate algodystrophy, which may slowly worsen for years with no warning signs. Treatment should be undertaken as early as possible to avoid later complications. This typically calls for painkillers, cortisone, calcitonin (a hormone used to treat osteoporosis), and other drugs in tablet or cream form. Smokers should make quitting a priority. This condition is also suited to injection therapy, which can help reduce the adverse effects of the sympathetic nervous system and the nerves that have become so hyperreactive. Alternative treatments, such as osteopathy, chiropractic, occupational therapy, electrotherapy, and acupuncture, as well as vitamin C supplements, can play a complementary role and help the patient get back to normal.

A patient of mine consulted with me for the algodystrophy she had been suffering for some ten months. She was experiencing a lot of pain in her forearm, feeling a burning sensation and spasmodic electric shocks. Despite her being heavily medicated—including taking one narcotic—the pain was incapacitating her day and night. Her skin had become extremely sensitive and subject to excessive sweating; even the feeling of her clothes or bedsheets against her skin aggravated the pain. The muscle mass in her arm had contracted and her hand and fingers were so tightly clenched, she couldn't pick anything up. She had tried a number of approaches, but the results had been lukewarm at best. The pain had started ten months earlier, following an injection in her shoulder.

First, I prescribed her an anti-inflammatory cream and a muscle and nerve relaxant. I then administered a painless injection to some acupuncture points and administered a local and regional anesthetic with a soothing anti-inflammatory agent to the nerve in her forearm. Three weeks later, the patient was able to use her hand again, the color of her skin was back to normal, and her pain had been reduced by 80 percent. After three weeks, I administered a second injection, and everything gradually returned to normal.

Sciatica

Sciatica is a term used to refer to pain affecting the sciatic nerve, which runs from the lower three lumbar vertebrae all the way down each leg to the ends of the toes. Depending on where the irritation occurs—in the third, fourth, or fifth lumbar vertebra (L3, L4, or L5)—sciatic pain can be felt in different parts of the leg corresponding to the height of the offending disc. For example, pain stemming from L3 will be felt in the front of the thigh. Most individuals suffering sciatic pain feel it in the thigh and calf, meaning that the issue lies with L4 or L5. These are the lowest and most frequently injured of the five lumbar vertebrae.

In many cases, sciatica may follow back pain. The pain may be due to a herniated disc, but often originates in the ligaments. The lumbosacral and sacroiliac (SI) ligaments play such an important role in the symptoms of this condition, which can be uncannily similar to those of disc-related sciatica.[24]

Muscle issues are another factor that can lead to sciatic pain, though somewhat less frequently. For example, myofascial pain syndrome may be to blame—in other words, the trigger points in the gluteal or piriformis muscles. The piriformis is a small, pyramid-shaped muscle deep in the buttock that connects to the sacrum. It can become tense and irritated, and the compression may eventually cause sciatic pain. It's also thought that certain muscles juxtaposed to the sciatic nerve can irritate the nerve when they contract, causing pain in the leg. Treating the piriformis muscles may eliminate this sciatic pain.[25]

I remember treating a patient who presented with pain in one leg and numbness that had persisted for two months because the muscles had contracted around the nerve. I administered a muscle relaxant injection and he looked at me completely astonished. He couldn't believe how quickly the pain had disappeared.

The patients I've treated this way describe feeling a tingling sensation, like heat spreading through the leg, followed a few minutes later by a sudden feeling that all the symptoms have faded away. When muscles contract around a nerve, it can cause a feeling similar to the pins and needles we feel in our leg when we're not sitting properly. It's bad enough having that feeling for a few minutes, so can you imagine having to live with it for days, weeks, or even months? Needless to say, it's extremely unpleasant. When the pressure is finally released, patients feel the same kind of relief as when we stretch a leg that's gone to sleep. Here the devil really is in the details: by taking the time to examine patients properly, doctors can put their finger on the anomaly and solve the problem, even if it has persisted for weeks or months on end.

Lastly, other possible causes of sciatic pain include osteoarthritis and disc space narrowing (not to be confused with a herniated disc). Disc space narrowing causes compression, which over time irritates the nerves—including the sciatic nerve. This phenomenon grows more frequent with age, but it can also be observed in young people who have experienced multiple trauma from sports such as mountain biking and snowmobiling, as repeatedly absorbing bumps in the trail can cause the discs in the spine to degenerate, become brittle, and crack.

Piriformis syndrome

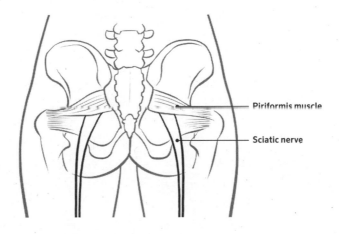

Piriformis muscle

Sciatic nerve

TREATMENT OPTIONS

When sciatica stems from the ligaments, treating the lumbosacral and sacroiliac (SI) ligaments will make the pain disappear. Treatment generally involves local injections, deep massage, or acupuncture.

Patients with myofascial pain syndrome and a knot in a gluteal or piriformis muscle will feel pain radiating down the leg. Deep massage or local injections will eliminate this sciatic pain.

If pain is brought on by muscles contracting around the sciatic nerve, injecting a muscle relaxant into the problematic muscle will automatically make the pain disappear.

Rehabilitation treatment with a physiotherapist, osteopath, or kinesiologist can then deliver long-term and problem-free results.

Sprains and pulled muscles

Sprains and pulled muscles frequently occur after spending too long in a poor posture—for example, by sitting for hours in front of a computer. Keeping the muscles at rest for an extended period can increase the risk of sprain or pulling, since sedentariness weakens the muscles.[26] Also, when we are under sustained stress, inflammatory poisons can saturate the muscles and create a state of constant tension without us realizing it.[27] Then, as soon as we solicit the slightest effort from our muscles, they can painfully spasm. This is why we can sometimes feel pain in our back or neck after the smallest false movement.

What's more, pain can suddenly appear and be very intense if we exercise without warming up first, or if our posture is incorrect. This pain can be more serious as it may result from a tear, causing what we call a pulled muscle. The pain can be immediately incapacitating, and if it occurs while running, for instance, the intense burning sensation can leave us limping all the way home.

When a muscle tears in the calf, a slight depression or swelling can be felt if a small hemorrhage (hematoma) forms around the tear. The areas of the body most commonly affected by stretched and pulled muscles are the limbs, and injuries are frequent during exercise.

More serious injuries can occur if the muscle tears. A ball-like mass can be seen where the shortened muscle is, and a deeper notch where the muscle has torn. The accessory muscles may compensate for any reduced mobility, however.

TREATMENT OPTIONS

Initial treatment calls for rest, ice, and compression bandages. If the injury is to the lower body, elevation of the leg will promote better circulation and proper drainage. Anti-inflammatories will be useful, but should only be taken after a few days to avoid hindering the initial inflammatory process as the body tries to repair the injury. This initial inflammation is actually beneficial because it stimulates the first stages of healing. During this acute phase (the first two days), massage is also contraindicated so as to avoid excessive bleeding. It's important to see a doctor, therapist, physiotherapist, osteopath, or chiropractor to confirm diagnosis and determine a course of treatment appropriate for the injury. Even if the muscle is torn, surgery will not necessarily be required: it all depends on the patient's age, as well as how strong their surrounding muscles are and how much these muscles can compensate for the weakness of the injured muscle.

Peripheral neuropathy

As its linguistic components—"neuro" and "pathos"—might suggest, peripheral neuropathy is essentially a form of suffering in the peripheral nervous system. The condition typically leads to a loss of sensitivity and a feeling of prickling and numbness in the feet or hands. Because sufferers no longer feel pain, they're at a greater risk of injuring or cutting themselves and developing infections. This form of neuropathy is most commonly associated with diabetics, as it affects 15 to 60 percent of individuals with diabetes. However, it may also be associated with alcoholism (often a lack of vitamin B), nutritional deficiencies, heavy-metal poisoning (such as mercury), some chemotherapy drugs, and sometimes even statins, which reduce levels of the protective antioxidant coenzyme Q10.

In diabetics, even if blood sugar is controlled relatively well, neuropathy is not a danger to be taken lightly. Like many other illnesses, diabetes causes a degeneration of the neuronal axons (extensions of the nerve cells), which, once attacked, will lead first to numbness, followed sometimes by dull aches or electric shock-like pain.

TREATMENT OPTIONS

While the usual painkillers can provide mixed relief, the danger of addiction is real, so it's best to pinpoint the cause before all else. Fortunately, alternative and complementary medicine hold a number of promising solutions that can resolve many of the causes of these peripheral nerve irregularities.

Alpha-lipoic acid can be a valuable ally in alleviating diabetic neuropathy (400–600 mg per day).[28] **Acetyl-L-carnitine, vitamin E, zinc, omega-3s, and L-glutamine** can also provide relief for neuropathies.

Acupuncture may be useful thanks to its therapeutic qualities, while **capsaicin** (cayenne pepper) in the form of a topical cream may relieve peripheral pain.

Transdermal medicated creams (compounded in pharmacies) can also be effective and promise no side effects.

Pulsed electromagnetic field (PEMF) therapy has also brought considerable relief to patients presenting with symptoms of peripheral neuropathy.[29] This technique is practiced by some chiropractors and physiotherapists.

Morton's neuroma

Another frequent neuropathy affecting the feet is Morton's neuroma. This affliction of the interdigital nerve on the sole of the foot just before the third and fourth toes can cause numbness and tingling in these two toes and the front part of the foot. If the condition persists, pain and sometimes electric shocks can be felt when walking. The pain can be so incapacitating, sufferers find themselves having to take off their shoe and massage their foot. As a general rule, wearing shoes that are too tight will aggravate the pain, which will tend to get even more incapacitating over time as the nerve is compressed by hypertrophy in the ligaments—this occurs for various mechanical reasons that aren't always clear.

TREATMENT OPTIONS

Appropriate footwear, massage, NSAIDs to relieve the pain, acupuncture, injections of various solutions to reduce inflammation and promote healing, physiotherapy, and osteopathy (with posturology) are all options that will usually solve the problem. In chronic cases, minor local surgery may eliminate the pain but will often lead to permanent loss of sensitivity in the toes.

Morton's neuroma

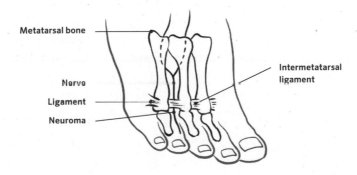

Metatarsal bone

Nerve

Ligament

Neuroma

Intermetatarsal ligament

Plantar fasciitis and heel spurs

Plantar fasciitis is an inflammatory condition affecting the sinewy ligament of the plantar fascia on the sole of the foot. It causes pain primarily in the heel, which can radiate into the rest of the foot. The pain tends to be worse when patients get up in the morning and take their first few steps out of bed. This is because the inflamed fascia contracts overnight, and the weight of standing on it in the morning painfully extends and stretches the fascia.

Often X-rays will show a small bony spur that has formed on the heel bone (calcaneus)—this is known as a heel spur. Most often, the spur is the result of too great a traction on the plantar fascia, which ends up depositing calcium particles at the attachment point of the calcaneus. Individuals with a heavier build or who have flat or hollow feet, as well as pregnant women, runners, and those who wear ill-fitting shoes or don't warm up properly before exercise, are the most at risk.

TREATMENT OPTIONS

It can be helpful to do some exercises to release the calf muscles, which will reduce tension on the calcaneus and on the fascia itself in turn. Avoid walking barefoot on hard surfaces. Ice massages and massages in general, as well as rolling a tennis ball over the sole of the foot, wearing shock-absorbing insoles, and trying injections and various other treatments, may all help if the problem persists. The key thing is to seek medical help sooner rather than later, because once a condition becomes chronic, it's always more complex and takes longer to treat.

Plantar fasciitis

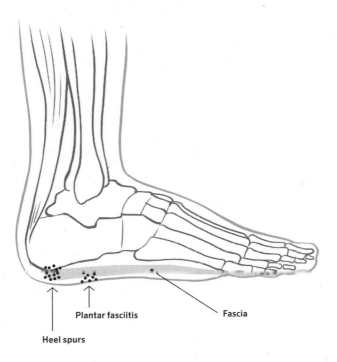

Heel spurs

Plantar fasciitis

Fascia

Acknowledgments

IIIIIIIIIIIIIIIIIIIIIIIIIIIIIIIIIIIIIIIIIIIIIIIIIIIIIIII

I WOULD LIKE TO thank my wife Carole, the instigator of my explo rations into pain, for her never-ending patience and support as this book came to be.

Thank you to Pascale at Les Éditions de l'Homme, my publisher in French, for encouraging me to write about pain.

Thank you to Véronique, my writing partner, who understood what I was trying to say and really grasped the ins and outs of pain. I'm thankful for all the dedication and research you put into these pages.

Thank you to my wonderful daughter-in-law Natasha, the pioneer who earned her stripes at the Institute for Functional Medicine (IFM) and made such a great contribution to the chapter on nutrition.

Thank you to my son Philippe, for his ongoing interest in overall health, his exercise and coaching talent, and his computer expertise.

Thank you to my son Simon, his wife Gabrielle, and especially their two daughters and twin boys, who would surely have liked to see a little more of their grandfather when he was busy writing.

Thank you to my patients, all six thousand plus of you. Throughout my forty-plus years of pain-focused medical practice, you have all helped me explore different treatment avenues around the world.

I would like to express my appreciation for the greatly inspiring medical experts I have met here in Canada and especially in the United States and Europe. Thank you for sharing your human knowledge and passion. I am especially grateful to the teachers of functional medicine at the IFM who weave together science and feeling to restore humans' vital energy in our often barren modern environment.

Finally, thank you to my life coach, DDD, for shedding more light and judgment on my understanding of the suffering we humans long to free ourselves from, so we can play a more active and conscious role in our destiny.

||||||||||||||||||||||||||||||||

TO LISTEN TO or watch free audio and video recordings that complement the information in this book, or find out more about the author's workshops and talks for the medical community and the general public, please visit drbrouillard.com.

Notes

‖‖

Introduction

1. T. M. A. Wijnhoven et al., "WHO European Childhood Obesity Surveillance
    Initiative: Health-Risk Behaviours on Nutrition and Physical Activity in
    6-9-Year-Old Schoolchildren," *Public Health Nutrition* 18, no. 17 (December
    2015): 3108-24; J. Lv et al., "Adherence to Healthy Lifestyle and Cardiovascular
    Diseases in the Chinese Population," *Journal of American College Cardiology* 69,
    no. 9 (March 7, 2017): 1116-25; O. J. Schiepers et al., "Lifestyle for Brain Health
    (LIBRA): A New Model for Dementia Prevention," *International Journal of Geri-
    atric Psychiatry* (February 28, 2017); R. Arena et al., "The Current Global State
    of Key Lifestyle Characteristics: Health and Economic Implications," *Progress
    in Cardiovascular Diseases* 59, no. 5 (March-April 2017): 422-29; J. J. Muros et
    al., "The Association between Healthy Lifestyle Behaviors and Health-Related
    Quality of Life among Adolescents," *Jornal de Pediatria (Rio Jornal)* (January 5,
    2017); Z. Wang et al., "Composite Protective Lifestyle Factors and Risk of Devel-
    oping Gastric Adenocarcinoma: The Singapore Chinese Health Study," *British
    Journal of Cancer* 116, no. 5 (February 28, 2017): 679-87; T. Kanagasabai and
    J. P. Chaput, "Sleep Duration and the Associated Cardiometabolic Risk Scores
    in Adults," *Sleep Health* 3, no. 3 (June 2017): 195-203; B. J. Arsenault and J. P.
    Després, "Cardiovascular Disease Prevention: Lifestyle Attenuation of Genetic
    Risk," *Nature Reviews Cardiology*, no. 14 (2017): 187-88; J. Hamer and E. Warner,
    "Lifestyle Modifications for Patients with Breast Cancer to Improve Prognosis
    and Optimize Overall Health," *Canadian Medical Association Journal* 189, no. 721

(February 2017): E268–74; R. S. Mazzeo, P. Cavanagh, W. J. Evans, et al., "Exercise and Physical Activity for Older Adults," *Medicine and Science in Sports and Exercise* 30, no. 6 (1998): 992–1008.

2. E. B. Dayoub, "Chronic Disease Prevalence and Healthy Lifestyle Behaviors among US Health Care Professionals," *Mayo Clinic Proceedings* 90, no. 12 (December 2015): 1659–62; R. F. Kushner and K. W. Sorensen, "Lifestyle Medicine: The Future of Chronic Disease Management," *Current Opinion in Endocrinology, Diabetes and Obesity* 20, no. 5 (October 2013): 389–95; J. J. Koopman and R. S. Kuipers, "From Arterial Ageing to Cardiovascular Disease," *The Lancet* 389, no. 10080 (April 2017): 1676–78; P. Elwood et al., "Healthy Lifestyles Reduce the Incidence of Chronic Diseases and Dementia: Evidence from the Caerphilly Cohort Study," *PloS One* 8, no. 12 (December 2013): e81877.

3. The Institute for Functional Medicine, "What Is Functional Medicine?" functionalmedicine.org/What_is_Functional_Medicine/AboutFM/. The functional medicine approach has been spearheaded and taught to thousands of doctors around the world by experts at the Institute for Functional Medicine (IFM) in Federal Way, WA. For the last twenty years, I have been fortunate to count some of the leading scientists and clinicians in this field as my personal mentors in functional medicine. Among these are Drs. David Jones, Jeffrey Bland, and Mark Hyman, who wrote the wonderful 800-page *Textbook of Functional Medicine*.

4. World Health Organization, "WHO Traditional Medicine Strategy: 2014–2023" (2013), apps.who.int/medicinedocs/documents/s21201en/s21201en.pdf.

5. J. H. Cyriax, *Slipped Disc*, Revised 2nd ed. (Aldershot, UK: Gower Press, 1975); Cyriax, *Massage, Manipulation and Local Anaesthesia* (London: Hamilton, 1941); Cyriax, *Textbook of Orthopaedic Medicine: Volume Two, Treatment by Manipulation, Massage and Injection*, 8th ed. (Philadelphia: The Williams & Wilkins Company, 1971); Cyriax, *Textbook of Orthopaedic Medicine: Diagnosis of Soft Tissue Lesions, Vol. 1*, 6th ed. (San Diego: Harcourt, 1975); Cyriax, *Textbook of Orthopaedic Medicine: Treatment by Manipulation, Massage and Injection, Vol. 2* (Kent, UK: Bailliere Tindall, 1980); Cyriax, *Illustrated Manual of Orthopaedic Medicine* (Kent, UK: Butterworth Heinemann, 1983); J. H. Cyriax and M. Coldham, *Textbook of Orthopaedic Medicine, Vol. 2: Treatment by Manipulation, Massage and Injection*, 11th ed. (Kent, UK: Bailliere Tindall, 1984).

6. R. Maigne, *J'ai mal au dos! Tout savoir pour s'en sortir* (Le Grand Livre du Mois, 1998); Maigne, *Douleurs d'origine vertébrale et traitements par manipulations* (Paris: Expansion scientifique française, 1977); Maigne, *Tout sur les*

manipulations vertébrales (Paris: Hachette, 1981); Maigne, *Mal de dos, mal du siècle* (Paris: Robert Laffont, 1992); Maigne, *Douleurs d'origine vertébrale: Comprendre, diagnostiquer et traiter* (Paris: Elsevier Masson, 2006); R. Maigne, R. Lescure, and R. Waghemacker, *Les Manipulations vertébrales* (Paris: Expansion scientifique française, 1961).

7. Quoted in Danny Raymond, "Auto-diagnostic en ligne: danger!" Agence Science Presse, *La Presse* (September 2, 2009).

Chapter 1: Understanding Pain

1. This definition from the International Association for the Study of Pain was first formulated in 1964 by Harold Merskey and quoted in a study published in *Pain* no. 6 (1979): 250.

2. R. Melzack and P. D. Wall, "Pain Mechanisms: A New Theory," *Science* 150, no. 3699 (November 19, 1965): 971-79.

3. S. A. Stratton, "Role of Endorphins in Pain Modulation," *Journal of Orthopaedics and Sports Physical Therapy* 3, no. 4 (1982): 200-205.

4. B. Fischer and E. Argento, "Prescription Opioid Related Misuse, Harms, Diversion and Interventions in Canada: A Review," *Pain Physician* 15, no. 3 (Supplement, July 1, 2012): ES191-203.

5. D. Schopflocher, R. Jovey, et al., "The Burden of Pain in Canada, Results of a Nanos Survey," *Pain Research and Management* (2010).

6. J. Dahlhamer, J. Lucas, C. Zelaya, et al., Centers for Disease Control and Prevention, "Prevalence of Chronic Pain and High-Impact Chronic Pain among Adults—United States, 2016," *Morbidity and Mortality Weekly Report* 67 (2018): 1001-1006. doi: dx.doi.org/10.15585/mmwr.mm6736a2External; D. Schopflocher, P. Taenzer, and R. Jovey, "The Prevalence of Chronic Pain in Canada," *Pain Research and Management* 16, no. 6 (Nov.-Dec. 2011): 445-50; L. Swain, G. Catlin, and M. P. Beaudet, "The National Population Health Survey—Its Longitudinal Nature," Statistics Canada, Health Reports 10, no. 4 (spring 1999), www150.statcan.gc.ca/n1/pub/82-003-x/1998004/article/4511-eng.pdf.

7. P. L. Ramage-Morin, "Chronic Pain in Canadian Seniors: Findings," *Health Reports* 19, no, 1 (2008), www150.statcan.gc.ca/n1/pub/82-003-x/2008001/article/10514/5002579-eng.htm; E. Chau, "1 in 5 Canadians Struggles with Chronic Pain," CBC News, April 30, 2014, cbc.ca/news/canada/british-columbia/1-in-5-canadians-struggles-with-chronic-pain-1.2622277.

8. Statistics Canada, *Rapports sur la santé* 7, no. 4.

9. D. J. Gaskin and P. Richard, "The Economic Costs of Pain in the United States," *The Journal of Pain* 13, no. 8 (2012): 715.

Chapter 3: Why Am I in Pain?

1. F. W. Booth et al., "Lack of Exercise Is a Major Cause of Chronic Diseases," *Comprehensive Physiology* 2, no. 2 (2012): 1143-211.

2. A. Arfè et al., "Non-Steroidal Anti-inflammatory Drugs and Risk of Heart Failure in Four European Countries: Nested Case-Control Study," *British Medical Journal*, no. 354 (2016): i4857.

3. K. B. Sondergaard et al., "Non-Steroidal Anti-inflammatory Drug Use Is Associated with Increased Risk of Out-of-Hospital Cardiac Arrest: A Nationwide Case-Time-Control Study," *European Heart Journal of Cardiovascular Pharmacotherapy* 3, no. 2 (2017): 100-107.

4. E. M. Quigley, "Gut Bacteria in Health and Disease," *Journal of Gastroenterology and Hepatology* 9, no. 9 (September 2013): 560-69.

5. H.-Y. Qin et al., "Impact of Psychological Stress on Irritable Bowel Syndrome," *World Journal of Gastroenterology* 20, no. 39 (October 21, 2014): 14126-31; S. Pellissier and B. Bonaz, "The Place of Stress and Emotions in the Irritable Bowel Syndrome," *Vitamins and Hormones*, no. 103 (2017): 327-54; S. M. O'Mahony, G. Clarke, T. G. Dinan, and J. F. Cryan, "Irritable Bowel Syndrome and Stress-Related Psychiatric Co-morbidities: Focus on Early Life Stress," *Handbook of Experimental Pharmacology*, no. 239 (2017): 219-46.

6. S. C. Bischoff et al., "Intestinal Permeability—A New Target for Disease Prevention and Therapy," *BMC Gastroenterology*, no. 14 (2014): 189; M. Campos, "Leaky Gut: What Is It, and What Does It Mean for You?" *Harvard Health Blog*, September 22, 2017, health.harvard.edu/blog/leaky-gut-what-is-it-and-what-does-it-mean-for-you-2017092212451; Q. Mu, J. Kirby, et al., "Leaky Gut as a Danger Signal for Autoimmune Diseases," *Frontiers in Immunology* (May 23, 2017), doi: 10.3389/fimmu.2017.00598.

7. J. A. Foster et al., "Gut Microbiota and Brain Function: An Evolving Field in Neuroscience," *International Journal of Neuropsychopharmacology* 19, no. 5 (May 2016): pyv114.

8. G. S. Hackett, *Ligament and Tendon Relaxation Treated by Prolotherapy* (Springfield, IL: Charles C. Thomas, 1956).

9. G. S. Hackett, "Referred Pain from Low Back Ligament Disability," *JAMA Surgery* (November 1956); T. Torstensson et al., "Referred Pain Patterns Provoked on Intra-pelvic Structures among Women with and without Chronic Pelvic Pain: A Descriptive Study," *PloS One* 10, no. 3 (2015): e0119542; D. Kurosawa, E. Murakami, and T. Aizawa, "Referred Pain Location Depends on the Affected Section of the Sacroiliac Joint," *European Spine Journal* 24, no. 3 (March 2015): 521–27; L, Arendt-Nielsen et al., "Basic Aspects of Musculoskeletal Pain: From Acute to Chronic Pain," *The Journal of Manual and Manipulative Therapy* 19, no. 4 (November 2011): 186–93.

10. R. P. McGovern and L. M. RobRoy, "Managing Ankle Ligament Sprains and Tears: Current Opinion," *Open Access Journal of Sports Medicine* 7 (2016): 33–42.

11. J. L. Zitnay et al., "Molecular Level Detection and Localization of Mechanical Damage in Collagen Enabled by Collagen Hybridizing Peptides," *Nature Communications,* no. 8 (2017): 14913.

12. E. Habibi et al., "Ergonomic Assessment of Musculoskeletal Disorders Risk among the Computer Users by Rapid Upper Limb Assessment Method," *International Journal of Environmental Health Engineering* 5 (2016): 15; O. P. Parry, P. Coenen, P. B. O'Sullivan, et al., "Workplace Interventions for Increasing Standing or Walking for Preventing Musculoskeletal Symptoms in Sedentary Workers," *Cochrane Database of Systematic Reviews* 1 (2017): CD012486; J. Wahlström, "Ergonomics, Musculoskeletal Disorders and Computer Work," *Occupational Medicine (London)* 55, no. 3 (2005): 168–76.

13. M. Osterweis, A. Kleinman, and D. Mechanic (eds.), *Pain and Disability: Clinical, Behavioral, and Public Policy Perspectives*, Institute of Medicine (US) Committee on Pain, Disability, and Chronic Illness Behavior (Washington, D.C.: National Academies Press, 1987); L. Ye-Seul et al., "The Dynamic Relationship between Emotional and Physical States: An Observational Study of Personal Health Records," *Neuropsychiatric Disease and Treatment* 13 (2017): 411–19; S. C. Segerstrom and G. E. Miller, "Psychological Stress and the Human Immune System: A Meta-analytic Study of 30 Years of Inquiry," *Psychological Bulletin* 130, no. 4 (July 2004): 601–30; *Healthy Lifestyle Stress Management,* Mayo Clinic, mayoclinic.org/healthy-lifestyle/stress-management/in-depth/stress/art-20046037.

14. E. L. Worthington, Jr., et al., "Forgiveness, Health, and Well-Being: A Review of Evidence for Emotional versus Decisional Forgiveness, Dispositional Forgivingness, and Reduced Unforgiveness," *Journal of Behavioral Medicine* 30 (2007): 291–302.

15. Committee on Health Care for Underserved Women, *Adult Manifestations of Childhood Sexual Abuse*, American Congress of Obstetricians and Gynecologists, Committee Opinion, no. 498 (August 2011), acog.org/Clinical-Guidance-and-Publications/Committee-Opinions/Committee-on-Health-Care-for-Underserved-Women/Adult-Manifestations-of-Childhood-Sexual-Abuse.

16. G. Devroede, *Ce que les maux de ventre disent de notre passé* (Paris: Éditions Payot, 2015).

17. G. B. J. Andersson, "Epidemiological Features of Chronic Low-Back Pain," *The Lancet* 354, no. 9178 (August 14, 1999): 581–85.

18. A. De Souzenelle, *Le symbolisme du corps humain* (Paris: Albin Michel, 2016); D. Miron, *Décodage psychosomatique des maladies* (Escalquens, France: Quintessence, 2007); P. Marty and N. Nicolaidis, *Psychosomatique* (Bègles, France: L'Esprit du Temps, 1996).

19. T. Svensson et al., "Psychological Stress and Risk of Incident Atrial Fibrillation in Men and Women with Known Atrial Fibrillation Genetic Risk Scores," *Scientific Reports* 7 (February 14, 2017): 42613.

Chapter 4: Pain Treatment Starts on Your Plate

1. E. Cohen, M. Cragg, J. deFonseka, A. Hite, et al., "Statistical Review of US Macronutrient Consumption Data, 1965–2011: Americans Have Been Following Dietary Guidelines, Coincident with the Rise in Obesity," *Nutrition* 31 (2015): 727–32.

2. A. F. Heini and R. L. Weinsier, "Divergent Trends in Obesity and Fat Intake Patterns: The American Paradox," *The American Journal of Medicine* 102 (1997): 259–64; W. C. Willett, "Overview and Perspective in Human Nutrition," *Asia Pacific Journal of Clinical Nutrition* 17 (2008): 1–4.

3. K. Ošancová, S. Hejda, and K. Zvolánková, "Dietary Fat and Dietary Sugar," *The Lancet* 285 (2015): 494.

4. Office of Disease Prevention and Health Promotion, "Cut Down on Added Sugars," *2015–2020 Dietary Guidelines for Americans*, health.gov/dietaryguidelines/2015/resources/DGA_Cut-Down-On-Added-Sugars.pdf.

5. M. Lenoir, F. Serre, L. Cantin, and S. H. Ahmed, "Intense Sweetness Surpasses Cocaine Reward," *PloS One* 2 (2007): 1–8.

6. G. S. Hotamisligil, P. Arner, J. F. Caro, R. L. Atkinson, and B. M. Spiegelman, "Increased Adipose Tissue Expression of Tumor Necrosis Factor-Alpha in Human

Obesity and Insulin Resistance," *The Journal of Clinical Investigation* 95 (1995): 2409-15; E. Sucurro, M. A. Marini, S. Frontoni, M. L. Hibal, et al., "Insulin Secretion in Metabolically Obese, but Normal Weight, and in Metabolically Healthy but Obese Individuals," *Obesity* 16 (2008); P. Dandona, A. Aljada, and A. Bandyopadhyay, "Inflammation: The Link between Insulin Resistance, Obesity and Diabetes," *Trends in Immunology* 25 (2014): 4-7.

7. M. Hyman, *Eat Fat, Get Thin* (New York: Little, Brown and Company, 2016).

8. E. M. El-Omar, K. Oien, A. El-Nujumi, D. Gillen, et al., "*Helicobacter Pylori* Infection and Chronic Gastric Acid Hyposecretion," *Gastroenterology* 113 (1997): 15-24; A. J. Smolka and M. L. Schubert, "*Helicobacter Pylori*-Induced Changes in Gastric Acid Secretion and Upper Gastrointestinal Diseases," in N. Tegtmeyer and S. Backert (eds.), *Molecular Pathogenesis and Signal Transduction by Helicobacter pylori* (Cham: Springer International Publishing, 2017): 227-52; G. Kelly, "Hydrochloric Acid: Physiological Functions and Clinical Implications," *Alternative Medicine Review* 2 (1997): 116-27; J. V. Wright and L. Lenard, *Why Stomach Acid Is Good for You: Natural Relief from Heartburn, Indigestion, Reflux and GERD* (London: M. Evans & Co., 2001); S. Ayazi, J. M. Leers, A. Oezcelik, E. Abate, et al., "Measurement of Gastric pH in Ambulatory Esophageal pH Monitoring," *Surgical Endoscopy* 23 (2009): 1968-73.

9. L. Mayer, "Mucosal immunity," *Pediatrics* 111, vol. 6, part 3 (June 2003): 1595-600; J. L. Round and S.K. Mazmanian, "The Gut Microbiota Shapes Intestinal Immune Responses during Health and Disease," *Nature Reviews Immunology* 9 (May 2009), 313-23.

10. R. E. Ley, P. J. Turnbaugh, S. Klein, and J. I. Gordon, "Microbial Ecology: Human Gut Microbes Associated with Obesity," *Nature* 444 (2006): 1022-23; P. J. Turnbaugh, R. E. Ley, M. A. Mahowald, V. Magrini, et al., "An Obesity Associated Gut Microbiome with Increased Capacity for Energy Harvest," *Nature* 444 (2006): 1027-1131; P. J. Turnbaugh, M. Hamady, T. Yatsunenko, et al., "A Core Gut Microbiome in Obese and Lean Twins," *Nature* 457 (2009): 480-84; Y. Kadooka, M. Sato, K. Imaizumi, et al., "Regulation of Abdominal Adiposity by Probiotics (*Lactobacillus Gasseri* SBT2055) in Adults with Obese Tendencies in a Randomized Controlled Trial," *European Journal of Clinical Nutrition* 64 (2010): 636-43; J. Annadora, J. Bruce-Keller, M. Salbaum, et al., "Obese-Type Gut Microbiota Induce Neurobehavioral Changes in the Absence of Obesity," *Society of Biological Psychiatry* 7 (2014): 1-9; O. A. Baothman, M. A. Zamzami, I. Taher, et al., "The Role of Gut Microbiota in the Development of Obesity and Diabetes," *Lipids in Health and Disease* 15 (2016): 1-8; M. Sanchez, C. Darimont, V. Drapeau, S. Emady-Azar, et al., "Effect of *Lactobacillus Rhamnosus* CGMCC1.3724

Supplementation on Weight Loss and Maintenance in Obese Men and Women," *British Journal of Nutrition* 111 (2014): 1507–19.

11. M. M. Grönlund, O. P. Lehtonen, E. Eerola, and P. Kero, "Fecal Microflora in Healthy Infants Born by Different Methods of Delivery: Permanent Changes in Intestinal Flora after Cesarean Delivery," *Journal of Pediatric Gastroenterology and Nutrition* 28, no. 1 (1999): 19–25; J. Penders et al., "Factors Influencing the Composition of the Intestinal Microbiota in Early Infancy," *Pediatrics* 118, no. 2 (August 2006): 511–21.

12. A. E. Wold and I. Adlerberth, "Breast Feeding and the Intestinal Microflora of the Infant—Implications for Protection against Infectious Diseases," *Advances in Experimental Medicine and Biology* 478 (2000): 77–93; F. Guaraldi and G. Salvatori, "Effect of Breast and Formula Feeding on Gut Microbiota Shaping in Newborns," *Frontiers in Cellular and Infection Microbiology* 2 (2012): 94.

13. J. Suez, T. Korem, D. Zeevi, et al., "Artificial Sweeteners Induce Glucose Intolerance by Altering the Gut Microbiota," *Nature* 514 (2014): 181–86.

14. J. L. Kuk and R. E. Brown, "Aspartame Intake is Associated with Greater Glucose Intolerance in Individuals with Obesity," *Applied Physiology, Nutrition, and Metabolism* 41 (2016): 795–98.

15. Centers for Disease Control and Prevention, *Antibiotic/Antimicrobial Resistance: Protecting the Food Supply*, published online November 15, 2016, cdc.gov/drug resistance/protecting_food-supply.html; R. Wei, F. Ge, S. Huang, M. Chen, and R. Wang, "Occurrence of Veterinary Antibiotics in Animal Wastewater and Surface Water around Farms in Jiangsu Province, China," *Chemosphere* 82, no. 10 (2011): 1408–14; Union of Concerned Scientists, "Prescription for Trouble: Using Antibiotics to Fatten Livestock," published online August 11, 2009, ucsusa .org/food_and_agriculture/our-failing-food-system/industrial-agriculture/ prescription-for-trouble.html#; World Health Organization, "Antimicrobial Resistance from Food Animals," published online March 7, 2008, who.int/ foodsafety/fs_management/No_02_Antimicrobial_Mar08_EN.pdf; World Health Organization, "WHO Publishes List of Bacteria for Which New Antibiotics are Urgently Needed," February 27, 2017, who.int/medicines/news/bacteria-antibiotics-needed/en/; M. J. Gilchrist, C. Greko, D. B. Wallinga, et al., "The Potential Role of Concentrated Animal Feeding Operations in Infectious Disease Epidemics and Antibiotic Resistance," *Environmental Health Perspectives* 115, no. 2: 313–16; M. E. Doyle, "Alternatives to Antibiotic Use for Growth Promotion in Animal Husbandry," Food Research Institute, University of Wisconsin–Madison, April 2001.

16. J. R. Biesiekierski, E. D. Newnham, P. M. Irving, et al., "Gluten Causes Gastrointestinal Symptoms in Subjects without Celiac Disease: A Double-Blind Randomized Placebo-Controlled Trial," *The American Journal of Gastroenterology* 106 (2011): 508–14; E. D. Newnham, "Does Gluten Cause Gastrointestinal Symptoms in Subjects without Coeliac Disease?" *Journal of Gastroenterology and Hepatology* 26 (2011): 132–34; S. L. Peters, J. R. Biesiekierski, G. W. Yelland, et al., "Randomised Clinical Trial: Gluten May Cause Depression in Subjects with Non-coeliac Gluten Sensitivity—An Exploratory Clinical Study," *Alimentary Pharmacology & Therapeutics* 39 (2014): 1104–12; P. Mansueto, A. D'Alcamo, A. Seidita, and A. Carroccio, "Food Allergy in Irritable Bowel Syndrome: The Case of Non-celiac Wheat Sensitivity," *World Journal of Gastroenterology: WJG* 21 (2015): 7089; A. Carroccio, P. Mansueto, and G. Iacono, "Non-celiac Wheat Sensitivity Diagnosed by Double-Blind Placebo-Controlled Challenge: Exploring a New Clinical Entity," *American Journal of Gastroenterology* 107 (2012): 1898–906.

17. A. Fasano and T. Shea-Donohue, "Mechanisms of Disease: The Role of Intestinal Barrier Function in the Pathogenesis of Gastrointestinal Autoimmune Diseases," *Natural Clinical Practice in Gastroenterology & Hepatology* 2 (2005): 416–22; M. Camilleri, K. Lasch, and W. Zhou, "Irritable Bowel Syndrome: Methods, Mechanisms, and Pathophysiology. The Confluence of Increased Permeability, Inflammation, and Pain in Irritable Bowel Syndrome," *American Journal of Physiology—Gastrointestinal and Liver Physiology* 303 (2012): G775–85; S. Ishihara, Y. Tada, N. Fukuba, A. Oka, et al., "Pathogenesis of Irritable Bowel Syndrome—Review Regarding Associated Infection and Immune Activation," *Digestion* 87 (2013): 204–11; A. C. Ford and N. J. Talley, "Mucosal Inflammation as a Potential Etiological Factor in Irritable Bowel Syndrome: A Systematic Review," *Journal of Gastroenterology* 46 (2011): 421–31; J. Walker, L. Dieleman, D. Mah, et al., "High Prevalence of Abnormal Gastrointestinal Permeability in Moderate-Severe Asthma," *Clinical & Investigative Medicine* 37 (2014): 53–57; A. Sapone, K. M. Lammers, V. Casolaro, et al., "Divergence of Gut Permeability and Mucosal Immune Gene Expression in Two Gluten-Associated Conditions: Celiac Disease and Gluten Sensitivity," *BMC Medicine* 9 (2011): 1–11.

18. W. Atkinson, T. A. Sheldon, N. Shaath, and P. J. Whorwell, "Food Elimination Based on IgG Antibodies in Irritable Bowel Syndrome: A Randomised Controlled Trial," *Gut* 53 (2004): 1459–64; S. Zar, M. J. Benson, and D. Kumar, "Food-Specific Serum IgG4 and IgE Titers to Common Food Antigens in Irritable Bowel Syndrome," *American Journal of Gastroenterology* 100 (2015): 1550–57; A. Sapone, K. M. Lammers, G. Mazzarella, et al., "Differential Mucosal IL-17

Expression in Two Gliadin-Induced Disorders: Gluten Sensitivity and the Auto-immune Enteropathy Celiac Disease," *International Archives of Allergy and Immunology* 152 (2009): 75–80.

19. P. A. Hayes, M. H. Fraher, and E. Quigley, "Irritable Bowel Syndrome: The Role of Food in Pathogenesis and Management," *Gastroenterology and Hepatology* 10 (2014): 164–74; R. Lever, C. MacDonald, P. Waugh, and T. Aitchison, "Randomised Controlled Trial of Advice on an Egg Exclusion Diet in Young Children with Atopic Eczema and Sensitivity to Eggs," *Pediatric Allergy and Immunology* 9 (1998): 13–19; N. Gonsalves, G. Y. Yang, B. Doerfler, et al., "Elimination Diet Effectively Treats Eosinophilic Esophagitis in Adults; Food Reintroduction Identifies Causative Factors," *Gastroenterology* 142 (2012): 1451–59.e1451; A. J. Lucendo, Á. Arias, J. González-Cervera, et al., "Empiric 6-Food Elimination Diet Induced and Maintained Prolonged Remission in Patients with Adult Eosinophilic Esophagitis: A Prospective Study on the Food Cause of the Disease," *Journal of Allergy and Clinical Immunology* 131 (2013): 797–804; V. A. Jones, E. Workman, A. H. Freeman, et al., "Crohn's Disease: Maintenance of Remission by Diet," *The Lancet* 326 (1985): 177–80; A. C. Brown and M. Roy, "Does Evidence Exist to Include Dietary Therapy in the Treatment of Crohn's Disease?" *Expert Review of Gastroenterology & Hepatology* 4 (2010): 191–215.

20. S. Carding, K. Verbeke, T. D. Vipond, et al., "Dysbiosis of the Gut Microbiota in Disease," *Microbial Ecology in Health and Disease* 26, no. 10 (2006): 3402/mehd .v26.26191.

21. A full list of references for Natasha Azrak's section can be found at drbrouillard .com.

22. C. B. Esselstyn, Jr., *Prevent and Reverse Heart Disease* (New York: Avery Publishing, 2008).

Chapter 5: Natural Pain-Relief Solutions

1. S. J. Lin, E. Ford, M. Haigis, et al., "Calorie Restriction Extends Yeast Life Span by Lowering the Level of NADH," *Genes & Development* 18 (2004): 12–16; J. A. Mattison et al., "Caloric Restriction Improves Health and Survival of Rhesus Monkeys," *Nature Communications*, published online January 17, 2017, nature .com/articles/ncomms14063#results.

2. M. Wei et al., "Fasting-Mimicking Diet and Markers/Risk Factors for Aging, Diabetes, Cancer, and Cardiovascular Disease," *Science Translational Medicine* 9, no. 377 (February 15, 2017), stm.sciencemag.org/content/9/377/eaai8700.

3. S. Tejpal, "Effect of Proteolytic Enzyme Bromelain on Pain and Swelling after Removal of Third Molars," *Journal of International Society of Preventive and Community Dentistry* 6, no. 3 (February 15, 2017): S197–204; B. Shivani et al., "Serratiopeptidase: A Systematic Review of the Existing Evidence," *International Journal of Surgery* 11, no. 3 (April 2013): 209–17; W. W, Bolten et al., "The Safety and Efficacy of an Enzyme Combination in Managing Knee Osteoarthritis Pain in Adults: A Randomized, Double-Blind, Placebo-Controlled Trial," *Arthritis*, published online January 31, 2015, doi: 10.1155/2015/251521.

4. C. Cal et al., "Role of Resveratrol in Prevention, Apoptose and Chemo-immuno-sensitizing Activities," *Current Medicinal Chemistry—Anti-Cancer Agents*, no. 2 (2003): 77–93.

5. *World Drug Report 2018* (United Nations publication, Sales No. E.18.XI.9), unodc .org/wdr2018/prelaunch/WDR18_Booklet_1_EXSUM.pdf.

6. Government of Canada, "Information for Health Care Professionals: Cannabis (Marihuana, Marijuana) and the Cannabinoids," last updated spring 2018, canada.ca/en/health-canada/services/drugs-medication/cannabis/information-medical-practitioners/information-health-care-professionals-cannabis-cannabinoids.html; National Academies of Sciences, Engineering, and Medicine, *The Health Effects of Cannabis and Cannabinoids: The Current State of Evidence and Recommendations for Research*, Washington, DC: The National Academies Press, 2017, doi.org/10.17226/24625.

7. Statista, "Quarterly Number of Medical Marijuana Clients Registered in Canada between April 2015 and September 2018," statista.com/statistics/603356/canadian-medical-marijuana-clients-registered-by-quarter/; ProCon.org, "Number of Legal Medical Marijuana Patients," medicalmarijuana.procon.org/view .resource.php?resourceID=005889.

8. D. I. Abrams, P. Couey, et al., "Cannabinoid-Opioid Interaction in Chronic Pain," *Clinical Pharmacology and Therapeutics* 90 (2011): 844–51; P. Lucas and Z. Walsh, "Medical Cannabis Access, Use, and Substitution for Prescription Opioids and Other Substances," *International Journal of Drug Policy* 42 (April 2017): 30–35, doi: 10.1016/j.drugpo.2017.01.011.

9. B. Wilsey, T. Marcotte, et al., "Low-Dose Vaporized Cannabis Significantly Improves Neuropathic Pain," *The Journal of Pain* 14 (2012): 136–48.

10. I. Tabata et al., "Effects of Moderate-Intensity Endurance and High-Intensity Intermittent Training on Anaerobic Capacity and VO2max," *Medicine & Science in Sports and Exercise*, no. 10 (1996): 1327–30.

11. F. Vatansever and M. R. Hamblin, "Far Infrared Radiation (FIR): Its Biological Effects and Medical Applications," *Photonics Lasers Medicine* 4 (November 1, 2012): 255–66; M. E. Sears et al., "Arsenic, Cadmium, Lead, and Mercury in Sweat: A Systematic Review," *Journal of Environmental Public Health*, published online February 22, 2012, doi: 10.1155/2012/184745; F. G. Oosterveld et al., "Infrared Sauna in Patients with Rheumatoid Arthritis and Ankylosing Spondylitis. A Pilot Study Showing Good Tolerance, Short-Term Improvement of Pain and Stiffness, and a Trend towards Long-Term Beneficial Effects," *Clinical Rheumatology*, no. 1 (January 28, 2009): 29–34.

12. "Alerte au mercure sur France 5: Les amalgames dentaires sont toujours utilisés malgré les risques pour la santé," *Huffington Post France*, February 1, 2015; updated October 5, 2016.

13. J. Mutter, "Is Dental Amalgam Safe for Humans? The Opinion of the Scientific Committee of the European Commission," *Journal of Occupational Medicine and Toxicology* 6, no. 2 (2011); A. O. Summers et al., "Mercury Released from Dental 'Silver' Fillings Provokes an Increase in Mercury- and Antibiotic-Resistant Bacteria in Oral and Intestinal Floras of Primates," *Antimicrobial Agents Chemotherapy* 37, no. 4 (April 1993): 825–34; K. G. Homme et al., "New Science Challenges Old Notion that Mercury Dental Amalgam Is Safe," *Biometals* 27, no. 1 (2014): 19–24.

14. Health Canada, "The Safety of Dental Amalgam," Government of Canada website, last modified February 5, 2009, canada.ca/en/health-canada/services/drugs-health-products/reports-publications/medical-devices/safety-dental-amalgam-health-canada-1996.html.

15. International Academy of Oral Medicine and Toxicology, "The Safe Mercury Amalgam Removal Technique (SMART)," IAOMT website, 2016, iaomt.org/safe-removal-amalgam-fillings/.

16. K. A. Ritchie et al., "Health and Neuropsychological Functioning of Dentists Exposed to Mercury," *Occupational and Environmental Medicine* 59 (2002): 287–93.

17. M. J. Vimy et al., "Maternal-Fetal Distribution of Mercury (203Hg) Released from Dental Amalgam Fillings," *American Journal of Physiology* 258 (April 1990): R939–45.

Chapter 6: Ways to Treat Pain

1. National Institute on Drug Abuse, "Overdose Death Rates," last revised January 2019, drugabuse.gov/related-topics/trends-statistics/overdose-death-rates;

Government of Canada, "National Report: Apparent Opioid-Related Deaths in Canada," June 2019, health-infobase.canada.ca/datalab/national-surveillance-opioid-mortality.html.

2. Government of Canada, "Fentanyl," last updated April 18, 2019, canada.ca/en/ health-canada/services/substance-use/controlled-illegal-drugs/fentanyl.html; Council on Foreign Relations, "The U.S. Opioid Epidemic," last updated January 17, 2019, cfr.org/backgrounder/us-opioid-epidemic.

3. J. G. Travell and D. G. Simons, *Myofascial Pain and Dysfunction: The Trigger Point Manual, vol. 1* (Philadelphia: Williams & Wilkins, 1983); J. G. Travell and D. G. Simons, *Myofascial Pain and Dysfunction: The Trigger Point Manual, vol. 2* (Philadelphia: Lippincott Williams & Wilkins, 1992).

4. R. A. Hauser, et al., "A Systematic Review of Dextrose Prolotherapy for Chronic Musculoskeletal Pain," *Clinical Medicine Insights: Arthritis and Musculoskeletal Disorders* 9 (2016): 139–59; R. A. Hauser and I. S. Sprague, "Outcomes of Prolotherapy in Chondromalacia Patella Patients: Improvements in Pain Level and Function," *Clinical Medicine Insights: Arthritis and Musculoskeletal Disorders* 7 (February 17, 2014): 13–20; A. M. Ada and F. Yavuz, "Treatment of a Medial Collateral Ligament Sprain Using Prolotherapy: A Case Study," *Alternative Therapies in Health and Medicine* 21, no. 4 (July–August 2015): 68–71.

5. T. M. Best et al., "A Systematic Review of Four Injection Therapies for Lateral Epicondylosis: Prolotherapy, Polidocanol, Whole Blood and Platelet Rich Plasma," *British Journal of Sports Medicine* 43, no. 7 (July 2009): 471–81.

6. A. J. Vickers, D. Phil, and K. Linde, "Acupuncture for Chronic Pain," *JAMA* 311, no. 9 (March 5, 2014): 955–56; S. A. Jayasuriya, *Clinical Acupuncture* (Sri Lanka: Chandrakanthi, 1985); L. S. W. Chu et al., *Acupuncture Manual, a Western Approach* (New York: Dekker, 1976).

7. T. I. Usichenko, V. P. Lysenyuk, M. H. Groth, and D. Pavlovic, "Detection of Ear Acupuncture Points by Measuring the Electrical Skin Resistance in Patients before, during and after Orthopedic Surgery Performed under General Anesthesia," *Acupuncture and Electrotherapeutic Research* 28, nos. 3–4 (2003): 167–73.

8. M. S. Markov, "Magnetic Field Therapy: A Review," *Electromagnetic Biology and Medicine* 26, no. 1 (2007): 1–23; B. Strauch et al., "Evidence-Based Use of Pulsed Electromagnetic Field Therapy in Clinical Plastic Surgery," *Aesthetic Surgery Journal* 2 (March–April 2009): 135–43; T. Iannitti et al., "Pulsed Electromagnetic Field Therapy for Management of Osteoarthritis-Related Pain, Stiffness and Physical Function: Clinical Experience in the Elderly," *Clinical Interventions in*

Aging 8 (2013): 1289–93; M. Vadalà et al., "Mechanisms and Therapeutic Applications of Electromagnetic Therapy in Parkinson's Disease," *Behavioral and Brain Functions* 11 (2015): 26; M. I. Weintraub and S. P. Cole, "Pulsed Magnetic Field Therapy in Refractory Neuropathic Pain Secondary to Peripheral Neuropathy: Electrodiagnostic Parameters—Pilot Study," *Neurorehabilittion and Neural Repair* 18, no. 1 (2004): 42–46.

9. R. Tarrasch et al., "The Effect of Reflexology on the Pain-Insomnia-Fatigue Disturbance Cluster of Breast Cancer Patients during Adjuvant Radiation Therapy," *Journal of Alternative and Complementary Medicine* 24, no. 1 (April 25, 2018): 62–68.

10. R. Nogier, *Introduction pratique à l'auriculomédecine, la photoperception cutanée* (Brussels: Haug International, 1993).

11. L. Rapolienè et al., "Stress and Fatigue Management Using Balneotherapy in a Short-Time Randomized Controlled Trial," *Evidence-Based Complementary and Alternative Medicine* (2016), doi: 10.1155/2016/9631684.

Chapter 7: The Psychology of Pain

1. I. Kirsch, "Antidepressants and the Placebo Effect," *Z Psychology* 222, no. 3 (2014): 128–34; A. Khan and W. A. Brown, "Antidepressants versus Placebo in Major Depression: An Overview," *World Psychiatry* 14, no. 3 (October 2015): 294–300.

2. A. Evrensel and M. E. Ceylan, "The Gut-Brain Axis: The Missing Link in Depression," *Clinical and Psychopharmacology Neurosciences* 13, no. 3 (December 2015): 239–44.

3. Josh Hafner, "What Happens if You Don't Sleep for 24 Hours? You're Basically Drunk," *USA TODAY*, published online March 22, 2017.

Chapter 8: Making Pain Easier to Live With

1. S. D. Kreibig, "Autonomic Nervous System Activity in Emotion: A Review," *Biological Psychology*, no. 84 (2010): 394–421; B. C. Sirois and M. M. Burg, "Negative Emotion and Coronary Heart Disease. A Review," *Behavior Modification* 27, no. 1 (January 2003): 83–102.

2. R. Veenhoven, "Healthy Happiness: Effects of Happiness on Physical Health and the Consequences for Preventive Health Care," *Journal of Happiness Studies*, no. 9 (2008): 449–69.

3. V. R. N. Menzies et al., "Effects of Guided Imagery on Outcomes of Pain, Functional Status, and Self-Efficacy in Persons Diagnosed with Fibromyalgia," *Journal of Alternative and Complementary Medicine* 12, no. 1 (January–February 2006): 23–30; C. J. Ackerman and B. Turkoski, "Using Guided Imagery to Reduce Pain and Anxiety," *Home Healthcare Nurse* 18, no. 8 (September 2000): 524–30; V. C. Tashjian, "Virtual Reality for Management of Pain in Hospitalized Patients: Results of a Controlled Trial," *JMIR Mental Health* 4, no. 1 (March 29, 2017): e9; M. P. Collins and L. F. Dunn, "The Effects of Meditation and Visual Imagery on an Immune System Disorder: Dermatomyositis," *Journal of Alternative and Complementary Medicine* 11, no. 2 (April 2005): 275–84.

4. Technique adapted from Simhananda, *Le yoga essentiel, science spirituelle* (Saint-Jean-sur-Richelieu, Quebec: Éditions Paume de Saint-Germain, 2010).

5. F. Zeidan et al., "Mindfulness Meditation-Related Pain Relief: Evidence for Unique Brain Mechanisms in the Regulation of Pain," *Neurosciences Letter* 520, no. 2 (June 29, 2012): 165–73; S. Banth and M. D. Ardebil, "Effectiveness of Mindfulness Meditation on Pain and Quality of Life of Patients with Chronic Low Back Pain," *Journal of Yoga* 8, no. 2 (July–December 2015): 128–33; P. La Cour and M. Petersen, "Effects of Mindfulness Meditation on Chronic Pain: A Randomized Controlled Trial," *Pain Medicine* 16, no. 4 (April 2015): 641–52.

6. J. W. Carson and F. J. Keefe, "Forgiveness and Chronic Low Back Pain: A Preliminary Study Examining the Relationship of Forgiveness to Pain, Anger, and Psychological Distress," *Journal of Pain* 6, no. 2 (February 2015): 84–91; E. Ricciardi et al., "How the Brain Heals Emotional Wounds: The Functional Neuroanatomy of Forgiveness," *Frontiers in Human Neurosciences*, no. 7 (2013): 839.

7. G. N. Fox et al., "Neural Correlates of Gratitude," *Frontiers in Psychology*, no. 6 (2015): 1491; R. A. Sansone and L. A. Sansone, "Gratitude and Well Being: The Benefits of Appreciation," *Psychiatry* (*Edgmont*) 7, no. 11 (2010): 18–22.

Appendix: Pain Guide

1. L. Yang et al., "A Possible Role of Intestinal Microbiota in the Pathogenesis of Ankylosing Spondylitis," *International Journal of Molecular Science* 17, no. 12 (December 2016): 2126; J. D. Forbes, G. Van Domselaar, and C. N. Bernstein, "The Gut Microbiota in Immune-Mediated Inflammatory Diseases," *Frontiers in Microbiology*, no. 7 (2016): 1081.

2. N. Tabibian et al., "Abdominal Adhesions: A Practical Review of an Often Overlooked Entity," *Annual Medical Surgery* (*London*), no. 15 (March 2017): 9–13.

3. D. S. Albrecht et al., "Differential Dopamine Function in Fibromyalgia," *Brain Imaging and Behavior* 10, no. 3 (September 2016): 829–39; D. J. Clauw and H. Ueda, "Summary of the Fibromyalgia Research Symposium 2016 in Nagasaki," *PAIN Reports* 2, no. 1 (January/February 2017): e582.

4. B. Sánchez-Domínguez et al., "Oxidative Stress, Mitochondrial Dysfunction and Inflammation, Common Events in Skin of Patients with Fibromyalgia," *Mitochondrion*, no. 21 (March 2015): 69–75; M. D. Cordero et al., "Oxidative Stress and Mitochondrial Dysfunction in Fibromyalgia," *Neuro Endocrinology Letters* 31, no. 2 (2010): 169–73.

5. B. Cagnie et al., "Central Sensitization in Fibromyalgia? A Systematic Review on Structural and Functional Brain MRI," *Seminars in Arthritis and Rheumatism* 44, no. 1 (August 2014): 68–75.

6. Centers for Disease Control and Prevention, "Fibromyalgia," last reviewed October 11, 2017, cdc.gov/arthritis/basics/fibromyalgia.htm; National Fibromyalgia Association, "Prevalence," 2018, fmaware.org/about-fibromyalgia/prevalence/.

7. "2012 Canadian Fibromyalgia Guidelines," Canadian Rheumatology Association website, rheum.ca/resources/publications/canadian-fibromyalgia-guidelines/.

8. B. G. Malatji et al., "A Diagnostic Biomarker Profile for Fibromyalgia Syndrome Based on an NMR Metabolomics Study of Selected Patients and Controls," *BMC Neurology*, no. 17 (2017): 88.

9. B. Gerdle, "Chronic Widespread Pain: Increased Glutamate and Lactate Concentrations in the Trapezius Muscle and Plasma," *Clinical Journal of Pain* 30, no. 5: 409–20.

10. K. Imbierowicz and U. T. Egle, "Childhood Adversities in Patients with Fibromyalgia and Somatoform Pain Disorder," *European Journal of Pain* 7, no. 2 (2003): 113–19.

11. J. Vas et al., "Acupuncture for Fibromyalgia in Primary Care: A Randomised Controlled Trial," *Acupuncture in Medicine (BMJ)* 34, no. 4 (February 15, 2016): 257–66, doi: 10.1136/acupmed-2015-010950.

12. C. Gaul, H. C. Diener, and U. Danesch (Migravent® Study Group), "Improvement of Migraine Symptoms with a Proprietary Supplement Containing Riboflavin, Magnesium and Q10: A Randomized, Placebo-Controlled, Double-Blind, Multicenter Trial," *Journal of Headache Pain*, no. 16 (2015): 516.

13. J. W. Olney, "Brain Lesions, Obesity, and Other Disturbances in Mice Treated with Monosodium Glutamate," *Science* 164, no. 3880 (May 9, 1969): 719–21.

14. K. J. Sherman et al., "Five-Week Outcomes from a Dosing Trial of Therapeutic Massage for Chronic Neck Pain," *Annals of Family Medicine* 12, no. 2 (March 2014): 112-20.

15. Y. Tanaka et al., "Cervical Roots as Origin of Pain in the Neck or Scapular Regions," *Spine* 31, no. 17 (August 1, 2016): E568-73.

16. Back Clinics of Canada, "What Is Whiplash?" backclinicsofcanada.ca/article/what-is-whiplash/; P. Tsoumpos et al., "Whiplash Injuries in Sports Activities: Clinical Outcome and Biomechanics," *British Journal of Sports Medicine* 47, no. 10 (April 2013): e3.

17. M. Fralick et al., "Association of Concussion with the Risk of Suicide: A Systematic Review and Meta-analysis," *JAMA Neurology* 76, no. 2 (2019): 144-51, doi:10.1001/jamaneurol.2018.3487.

18. M. C. Thompson et al., "US Pediatric Injuries Involving Amusement Rides, 1990-2010," *Clinical Pediatrics* 52, no. 5 (May 1, 2013): 443-40. doi: 10.1177/0009922813476341.

19. H. R. Weiss et al., "Postural Rehabilitation for Adolescent Idiopathic Scoliosis during Growth," *Asian Spine Journal* 10, no. 3 (June 2016): 570-81.

20. W. Brinjikji et al., "Systematic Literature Review of Imaging Features of Spinal Degeneration in Asymptomatic Populations," *AJNR American Journal of Neuroradiology* 36, no. 4 (April 2015): 811-16.

21. A. Vaquero-Picado et al., "Lateral Epicondylitis of the Elbow," *EFORT Open Reviews* 1, no. 11 (November 2016): 391-97.

22. S. Swapneel Karne and N. Sudhakar Bhalerao, "Carpal Tunnel Syndrome in Hypothyroidism," *Journal of Clinical and Diagnostic Research* 10, no. 2: OC36-38.

23. E. L. Goh et al., "Complex Regional Pain Syndrome: A Recent Update," *Burns Trauma* 5 (2017): 2.

24. E. Murakami et al., "Leg Symptoms Associated with Sacroiliac Joint Disorder and Related Pain," *Clinical Neurology and Neurosurgery* 157 (June 2017): 55-58.

25. L. A. Boyajian-O'Neill et al., "Diagnosis and Management of Piriformis Syndrome: An Osteopathic Approach," *The Journal of the American Osteopathic Association* 108 (November 2008): 657-64.

26. S. D. Stovitz and R. J. Johnson, "'Underuse' as a Cause for Musculoskeletal Injuries: Is It Time that We Started Reframing Our Message?" *British Journal of Sports Medicine* 40, no. 9 (September 2006): 738-39.

27. K. M. Poornima et al., "Study of the Effect of Stress on Skeletal Muscle Function in Geriatrics," *Journal of Clinical and Diagnostic Research* 8, no. 1 (January 2014): 8–9.

28. N. Vallianou et al., "Alpha-Lipoic Acid and Diabetic Neuropathy," *Reviews in Diabetic Studies* 6, no. 4 (Winter 2009): 230–36.

29. K. Suszynski, W. Marcol, and D. Górka, "Physiotherapeutic Techniques Used in the Management of Patients with Peripheral Nerve Injuries," *Neural Regeneration Research* 10 (2015): 1770–72.

Index

About the Author

|||||||||||||||||||||||||||||||||||||||||||||||||||||||||||||

DR. GAÉTAN BROUILLARD is a bestselling author who writes about alternative approaches to health. After starting his career as an emergency physician in Montreal, he worked as a clinical instructor for thirty-five years alongside his private medical practice. An expert in the treatment of chronic pain, he practices preventive and functional medicine and works acupuncture, naturopathy, osteopathy, and hypnotherapy into his clinical approach. As a conference speaker and author, Dr. Brouillard promotes a multifaceted approach to health centered on the person, not the problem. Drawing on the principles of holistic and integrative medicine, he explains just how instrumental a role lifestyle and environment have to play when it comes to our health.